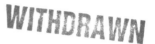
The Plant-Based Workplace

*Add Profits, Engage Employees and
Save the Planet*

Gigi Carter

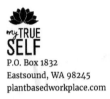

P.O. Box 1832
Eastsound, WA 98245
plantbasedworkplace.com

LinkedIn: www.linkedin.com/in/gigicarter/
Twitter: @GigiMyTrueSelf
Website: mytrueself.com

PUBLISHER: Gigi Carter through Amazon Publishing
EDITOR: Loretta Rafey
COVER DESIGN: Erika at EA5Designs

Every effort has been made to correctly attribute all material reproduced and to ensure the accuracy of the information contained throughout this book. If any error has been made unwittingly, we will be happy to correct it in future editions.

WHAT THE EXPERTS SAY ABOUT
The Plant-Based Workplace

"What a beautifully written and timely book. Drawing upon her personal health journey as well as her years in the corporate world, Gigi Carter has filled *The Plant-Based Workplace* with cogent analysis and practical action plans to help companies large and small use wiser nutrition choices to improve their employees' health and their company's bottom lines - and, oh yes, save Planet Earth from disaster at the same time. Thank you, Gigi Carter, for shining this much needed light on the heretofore unexplored - yet essential - role the business world can play in solving our nation's health and environmental challenges. After all, improving our health and healing our planet is everyone's business, and *The Plant-Based Workplace* gives us the blueprint to accomplish both goals - so I can most highly recommend this insightful and well-written book."

Michael Klaper, MD

"Gigi Carter brings a powerful new voice to the healthy food movement. Her background in both corporate America and nutrition science enables her to present a practical and compelling roadmap for the business community to improve the health and productivity of their workers, lower healthcare costs, and contribute to a cleaner and more sustainable environment."

Paul Simon, MD, MPH
Adjunct Professor, UCLA Fielding School of Public Health

"*The Plant-Based Workplace* is a must read! Gigi Carter introduces a revolutionary, thoughtful, and progressive blueprint for businesses that will inspire organizational change, create healthier people, and regenerate the environment through sincere resource stewardship. It is the true win-win-win scenario for every stakeholder and the future that we will leave to our children."

Scott Stoll, MD, FABPMR
Co-Founder and Chairman Plantrician Project
Co-Founder International Plant Based Nutrition Healthcare Conference
Author, Olympian, Speaker

"Gigi Carter provides a convincing argument with data that a plant-based diet in the workplace is not only the right thing to do from an employee health perspective... but also from the company's bottom line perspective. This book is a blue print for any business leader..."

Jay Iyengar
SVP, Chief Innovation & Technology Officer, Xylem Inc.

Dedicated to those who find true freedom in taking control of their health.

FOREWORD

In my 30 years of practicing medicine focused on preventive cardiology, there have been amazing advances. I remember the day long ago when I first heard of stents, then placed one in a patient's heart artery, and witnessed the miracle of technology. It didn't end there. My care of patients was bolstered by better medications by mouth or injection, operations done through small incisions and scopes, and even replacing heart valves through tiny catheters previously unimaginable.

Despite the marvel and pride to have witnessed and participated in these advances, the goal of caring for patients to improve their quality and quantity of life, and to do so in a manner responsible to the economy, has faltered. In the USA we spend more dollars on health than any other country and get only average care by most estimates in return. Lifespan is no longer going up, and the last few decades of life are often a battle with the chronic diseases of the heart, cancer, diabetes, failing joints and failing minds. Another term, our healthspan, is not going up and seems to be shortening for many despite all of these advances.

In my role as director of preventive cardiology and cardiac rehabilitation at two major hospital systems in Detroit in the past, as well as Director of Employee Wellness for over 10,000 workers, I participated firsthand in efforts to provide the best medical care of all types but saw that the efforts were usually on acute care, patching people back together but not really changing the root cause of the problem. Indeed, decades ago English physician Dennis Burkitt, MD, commented that health care is like a waterfall. People keep falling off the edge, into the water, get all banged up, and the medical system is there to efficiently put them together as best as possible. Dr. Burkitt asked the most important question however, what if we could keep people from going over the edge? What if we could put up a fence and prevent the injury in the first place?

Gigi Carter asks that same question in *The Plant-Based Workplace*. She has that combination of decades in corporate management and a recent journey into the sphere of health and wellness. It is like Pandora's Box to ask the question, is there a better way to live your lives in terms of diet and fitness to optimize our chances of being healthy, performing at our best, and not needing medication and surgery to get by? Just sitting down and watching the hit documentary *Forks Over Knives* for 75 minutes can blow away formed paradigms that diseases are managed. Why not reverse them? Better yet, why not prevent them? And why not use one of the most cost-effective strategies at home and at work, food, to meet those goals?

While there are many books on plant-based diets, the application to the workplace has been studied and shown to be effective but have not been the basis for a simple but impactful book to help human resource and C suite managers. I believe Ms. Carter has filled that need with this book. Chapters 1-6 provide a thorough and accurate recounting of the nature of chronic disease that impact the workforce and cost billions of dollars and so much pain and grief. The facts are available to all in referenced medical articles but are made accessible and practical in these chapters. Of interest, few treatises extend to the issue of the environmental impact of our food choices. While many companies might proudly have a recycling and composting effort, the power of a plant-based diet at work on the development of greenhouse gases and on water and air quality has not been stressed but is critical to consider.

Chapters 7-11 bring this information into focus for businesses. It has been shown that cafeterias, food truck providers, and vending machine options can be made healthy and plant-based and have an impact on the physical and emotional well-being of corporations. GEICO in suburban Washington, D.C., for example, participated in a trial comparing the healthy choices at some sites to the standard option at other sites, and found much benefit for their workers.

Is a plant-based approach too "radical" for a business? There is a momentum developing with high profile actors (Beyoncé) athletes (Kyrie Irving), politicians (Cory Booker), and physicians (me!) adopting plant diets and reporting improved performance and health. A leadership team presenting simple substitutions from beef to bean chili, and from pork to plant sausages, can start the movement with hardly a whimper or cost. Yet, businesses have so much to gain by a workforce that feels better, feels lighter, is less medicated, and shows up to work more often and in better spirits.

I believe *The Plant-Based Workplace* can be the basis of a successful and cost-effective program at any business and lead to a better workplace, a healthier workforce, and a more effective corporation. I am grateful that Ms. Carter put these important ideas into a book for all to consider and implement.

Joel Kahn, MD, FACC
Founder, Kahn Center for Cardiac Longevity
Clinical Professor, Wayne State University School of Medicine
drjoelkahn.com

CONTENTS

INTRODUCTION

A lthough my own wellness journey required several years to take root, I officially embarked on the plant-based journey in 2012. I was 41 years old and had grown tired of periodically detoxing due to a diet I mistakenly thought was healthy. The crucial shift occurred when I became aware of what is known as a "whole-food, plant-based" diet. Now, the word "diet" sometimes has the negative connotation of a capricious fad; sort of an overly ambitious New Year's resolution that lasts but a few weeks before giving way to the same old indulgences. But the definition of "diet" is simply what a person habitually eats. The plant-based diet caught my attention because I noticed I felt best during and following the detox regimens I tried, when I was only eating vegetables and fruits. Like many who transition to a whole-food, plant-based diet, I experienced increased energy levels and improved mental clarity. My bloodwork was no longer considered borderline after physician visits. My LDL (bad) cholesterol and triglycerides dropped more than 23% over the course of just a few months, and I started cycling. By 2014, I was in full plant-based athletic mode, having taken up bike racing and immersing myself in plant-based nutrition research. I competed and won two ultra-distance races: the RAAM 200 Florida Challenge in November 2014 and Bessie's Creek 24 in April 2015. At the age of 46, I continue to compete in Category 3 road bike racing. I even became the board president and team manager of the all-women's Nunchuck Bunnies bike racing team.

I acquired knowledge about the impact large-scale animal agriculture has on the environment as I was learning more about the nutritional benefits of a plant-based diet. The first report I read was "Livestock's Long Shadow" from the Food and Agriculture Organization of the United Nations, published in 2006. It is worth pointing out that here I was reading it seven years after its release. Was this old news? Why hadn't I heard about it sooner? The UN report comprehensively explained that animal agriculture is the largest contributor to greenhouse gases, eclipsing even the transportation sector. From an article in National Geographic and the National Oceanic and Atmospheric Administration, I learned how nitrogen discharge from factory farms of the Central and Midwestern United States was flowing into the Mississippi River and then enriching the Gulf of Mexico with excess nutrients. This process, known as "eutrophication," feeds algal blooms that pull oxygen from the water for photosynthesis. I learned that this oxygen loss creates "dead zones" that fish and other wildlife are subsequently unable to inhabit. This new knowledge disturbed me, and the once abstract nature of our food system became one of personal concern.

The positive life changes I experienced through dietary improvements and increased physical activity, along with my growing consciousness of the environmental implications of animal agriculture, motivated me to share what I learned with my broader work family. I pitched the idea of making comprehensive changes to the workplace food environment, but soon realized that implementing this kind of systemic change is bigger than any one person – even one in a leadership position – at a large multinational company can make. After 22 years of working my way up the ladder to various corporate management and leadership positions, I took a hiatus to pursue a master's degree in Nutrition Sciences with a focus on lifestyle management and disease prevention. I am now a licensed nutritionist, with training in plant-based nutrition, as well as a certified personal trainer. In this book I draw on several additional aspects of my multidisciplinary background: finance, process improvement (lean and six sigma), operations management, plus project and program management. The genesis of this book comes from my desire to help people, solve business problems, and conserve our shared global ecosystem – this truly is the trifecta! My book provides the necessary business case for employers to implement a plant-based workplace plan that will not only improve profits and employee health outcomes, but also establish more environmentally sustainable practices. How gratifying it will be to inspire the creation of workplace food environments that help extend and improve employees' quality of life while enhancing profits and leaving a lighter environmental footprint.

First, a few points about terminology. For the sake of simplicity, I use the descriptor "American" to identify the population of people residing in the United States of America. When referring to chronic diseases and conditions, I intentionally use phrases like "person with obesity" or "person with diabetes" and avoid using "obese person" or "diabetic" to emphasize that these are disease conditions that should not be used to erroneously label a whole person. The public health and medical community customarily use the phrase "having overweight and obesity" to describe people whose weights fall above what are considered healthy thresholds. For the sake of linguistic flow, I instead use the phrase "having excessive weight and obesity." In the chapters related to health and disease, I use the term "environment" to describe the surroundings or conditions in which a person operates. However, I also use the term "environment" in subsequent parts of this book pertaining to the ecosystem, environmental footprints, and sustainability. This practice is in keeping with the ecological science perspective that the human environment is equivalent to any other ecological environment. Finally, I use the term "plant-based" somewhat broadly. While my personal preference is for a whole-food, plant-based vegan diet, I also include in this plant-based continuum the DASH and Mediterranean diets, both of which are largely plant-based but also include small portions of animal products. Finally, I occasionally describe certain foods as either "healthy" or "unhealthy." When I refer to a food as healthy, I base this assessment on the following criteria: the food is nutrient-dense (rich in vitamins, minerals, antioxidants, and phytochemicals) and something health experts say we should eat more of. Foods I refer to as unhealthy are, by contrast, those that are calorically-dense and that health experts say we should limit in our diets or avoid. I make these individual assessments with the awareness that overall dietary patterns are more important than overemphasizing individual foods. Indeed, it is the sum of individual foods that makes up the dietary pattern.

This book comprises three main sections:

(1) What the medical literature says about links among lifestyle, environment, and chronic diseases, as well as what prevents (or reverses) these diseases. This section also explores scientific literature on the best food system sustainability practices for a growing population.

(2) The business case for implementing a plant-based workplace, from both a financial perspective and from the vantage point of ethical rationale. Namely, what poor employee health costs employers in terms of medical expenses and the reduced productivity associated with absenteeism and presenteeism. This is presented alongside the ethical rationale for a plant-based

workplace as a socially responsible practice that builds social capital with employees, customers, and other stakeholders.

(3) A change model and practical strategies any organization can apply to engage employees in the implementation of a plant-based workplace.

This book wraps up by challenging you, the reader, to make it personal. After all, people's lives are literally at stake, and being a visible, innovative leader may not only protect lives, but also guarantee the long-term social capital and financial sustainability of the entire organization.

SECTION I: THE LITERATURE

"All truth passes through three stages. First, it is ridiculed. Second, it is violently opposed. Third, it is accepted as being self-evident."

ARTHUR SCHOPENHAUER,
PHILOSOPHER (1788-1860)

1 | THE PREPONDERANCE OF EVIDENCE FOR INDIVIDUAL AND PLANETARY HEALTH

Health is conventionally defined as "the state of being free from illness or injury."[1] Many companies interpret this definition from an acute standpoint – meaning those abrupt incidents that require immediate first aid or emergency medical care, such as a surface cut to the skin, a broken bone, loss of limb, or loss of life. Most companies have Health and Safety policies, procedures, and workplace instructions that aim to minimize and respond to these types of events. Furthermore, companies implement safeguards in the form of hardhats, machine guarding, steel toe shoes, safety glasses, gloves and earmuffs to minimize the possibility of these injuries occurring. However, chronic disease threats are largely absent from company policies and protocols, even though chronic diseases make up over 80% of American healthcare costs and affect half of the country's adult population.[2] Perhaps disease prevention protocols are absent from company policies because companies don't believe their workplace environment is a factor in employee chronic diseases. Companies might believe that disease prevention is a personal matter an employee takes up with his or her physician, family and loved ones. But what if companies *do* play a fundamental role in promoting either health or disease?

Chronic diseases are non-communicable conditions or illnesses that progress slowly over time. The Centers for Disease Control and Prevention (CDC) includes heart disease, stroke, cancer, type 2 diabetes, obesity, and arthritis as chronic diseases and considers these conditions to be the most common, costly and largely preventable of all American health conditions.[2] Since chronic diseases are less salient than acute illnesses and injuries, it seems many companies do not consider the fiscal impact of employee chronic diseases on healthcare costs, productivity losses, and workers compensation claims. Exploring parallels with other types of workplace safety standards can illuminate this blind spot. For example, I often wonder why a manager or team leader calls a "safety stand-down" when a factory worker incurs a deep skin cut requiring sutures, in which all staff convene to discuss what happened. A "root cause and corrective action" process is initiated to determine what could be done to prevent similar situations in the future. However, when an employee has chest pains that require emergency medical transport, aside from the slight disruption of curious coworkers wondering why their colleague John is being carried away on a stretcher, no one thinks to initiate corrective action. No root workplace cause is determined, and no safety protocols are developed or implemented. Instead, it's back to work as usual. Why is that? Maybe it's because we take for granted that John's condition is rooted in his personal life and has nothing to do with workplace environmental conditions. However, I contend that many companies play an unwitting role in contributing to John's chronic disease through the workplace food environment.

Employees spend more than half of their waking life at work. According to Gallup, full-time employees in the United States work an average of 47 hours per week and about four in 10 say they work at least 50 hours per week.[3]   Employees who go to brick and mortar factories or office buildings often rely on cafeterias, workplace vending machines, and kiosks for one or more meals per day. Workplace food venues are an important service to employees, and I am calling on companies to apply more actively engaged scrutiny of the nutritional standards in these venues.

A study conducted by the Center for Science in the Public Interest, a nonprofit consumer advocacy group, found that of the 853 vending machines their researchers assessed, "only 5% of vended foods were healthy options, such as fruits, vegetables, or nuts."[4]   The nutritional quality of foods served in workplace cafeterias varies greatly depending on the city and community. Another study used data from 623 hospital employees who took a health risk assessment to determine if their awareness of personal elevated cholesterol levels changed subsequent food choice behaviors.[5] The researchers found that over the 15-week period following communication of participant bloodwork results, participants reduced their weekly food expenditures by 10-15%, and slightly increased (about 2-3%) spending on healthy food options in the workplace cafeteria.[5] Of particular relevance to the subject of this book is that even in a large regional medical center, where one would expect to see solely healthy foods, only 40% of the foods participants chose were considered healthy by nutritional criteria of the research team. Even in a hospital setting where a logical person would expect to see not only 100% healthy food options, but also higher-than-average nutritional awareness in the employee population, the results of no significant change in the employees' cholesterol levels after 15 weeks speaks to why the current corporate wellness model of "having some healthy options" does not work!

We all know people who pack their own lunches because they are trying to eat healthier, and whose on-site workplace food options are not helpful to them in achieving this health goal. Why are such people burdened with the extra work of packing their own lunches? Shouldn't this scenario be inverted such that unhealthy eating choices are the ones that require extra work? Shouldn't workplace food venues be designed using principles of behavioral economics (that applies psychology to economic decision making) to encourage healthy workplace eating?

The Health Belief Model is a psychological model that "addresses the individual's perceptions of the threat posed by a health problem (susceptibility, severity), the benefits of avoiding the threat and factors influencing the decision to act (barriers, cues to action and self-efficacy)."[6] The Health Belief Model is often touted as one of the key behavior change models for making lifestyle changes, such as smoking cessation, starting an exercise routine, or improving dietary nutrition. Under this model, what determines whether an individual successfully makes the change is the "perceived barriers" construct. If an individual seeks to implement a change but perceives a barrier too great to overcome, or feels there are too many small barriers to endure, the change won't happen. A 2017 study looks at perceived barriers to healthy workplace eating among people with obesity.[7] The results show that the top two perceived barriers to healthy eating are: (a) convenience and lack of self-control, and (b) lack of access to healthy foods.[7] If companies only offered healthy choices, would these barriers go away? In removing these barriers, would there be a reduction in the obesity rates?

The medical connection between food and health is widely established and dates as far back as 400 B.C., when Greek physician and father of medicine Hippocrates is said to have advised: "Let food be thy medicine and medicine be thy food." Over the past several decades, countless studies have looked at the role foods play in promoting health or disease. But what exactly is "healthy?" If health is a state in which one is free from illness, the preponderance of evidence supports that eating a diet rich in varied, plant-based whole foods will prevent most chronic diseases. I will explore this assertion further with additional evidence in later chapters.

The 2006 United Nations Food and Agriculture Organization report states that the livestock industry emits more greenhouse gases than the transportation sector; and its strain on water resources, combined with land degradation effects and threats to biodiversity, could be cataclysmic.[8, 9] With a global population projected to reach 9.8 billion by the year 2050[10], the evidence points to warming temperatures and greater food insecurity. The current model of animal agriculture is just not sustainable. Therefore, we need to consider from where we source our food. With this in mind, the adoption of a plant-based dietary pattern is our best option, because it uses fewer land and water resources and lessens the threat to biodiversity.

Throughout this book, I make assertions and claims based on the strength of the available scientific research findings. The rigor of the evidence related to diet and human health varies based on study design, with the strongest evidence found first in experimental studies, and second in observational studies.

Experimental study designs, most notably randomized controlled trials, are typically the strongest evidence because they enable a researcher to most persuasively establish "cause and effect." In these studies, there are typically two randomized groups of subjects, one group is exposed to the intervention and the other (control) group is not exposed to the intervention, or may be given a placebo, a "dummy" intervention presumed to have no effect on the variable of interest. With true randomization and designs that address both internal and external factors, researchers can establish baseline measurements, implement the intervention, and then measure the effects of both the intervention and control groups. Using these data, researchers draw conclusions about statistically significant causal relationships between variables to explain some phenomenon. Oftentimes, researchers take several randomized controlled trials and homogenize the results through a funneling process to draw a general conclusion about what the pool of studies found. These are referred to as systematic reviews and meta-analysis study designs.

Observational study designs include epidemiological (or population-wide), cross-sectional, case-control, and cohort studies, and are limited in being able to establish cause and effect but can be powerful in terms of guiding further research activities in specific areas. These observational studies often look at correlations and associations between different variables. For example, many people subscribe to the theory that a company with the best and brightest talent is also among the highest performing companies in their competitive market. While there is evidence to support a correlation between these two variables, without a well-designed randomized controlled trial, researchers cannot establish a causal relationship between having the best and brightest talent and highest performance among a peer group of companies. Even if there was a clearly established definition of what "best and brightest talent" means, the presence of other confounding variables can influence the outcome, such that no causal relationship can be asserted with confidence. Systematic reviews and meta-analysis studies also apply to observational studies, whereby researchers pool several different studies on the same or a closely related subject and try to draw broader conclusions about the results.

Animal studies are often used by scientists because their subjects are living creatures similar enough to humans to be experimented on for the sake of advancing scientific understanding of what may be applicable to humans without exposing humans to potential harms. Animal studies are considered "weaker" than experimental and observational studies of actual human subjects since animals do not have the exact same physiology as humans. However, these studies can help scientists focus further research efforts in subsequent human studies.

Finally, I provide personal anecdotes, opinions, and editorials in selected parts of this book to provide real world contexts and draw the reader into personally connecting with certain concepts and theories established in the various study designs I explore. These personal insights should not be taken as scientific evidence, but rather as inspiration or qualitative insight to inspire meaningful transformation. In keeping with the spirit of John Kotter and Daniel Cohen's best-selling *The Heart of Change*, appealing to the heart is, after all, the most effective driver of change. [11]

Before diving into the scientific studies on obesity, I want to share an anecdote from my days as an operations manager of an aerospace manufacturing plant in Mississippi. I was sitting in my office going through emails when a production employee stopped by. He had a worried look on his face as he told me that his father, who suffered from type 2 diabetes, would soon undergo another amputation. The employee wasn't asking me for anything; he just needed someone in management to care about his situation and listen. He lamented that his father wasn't taking decent care of himself. The family doctor had informed him that his father would likely lose not only a foot but possibly part of a leg due to the advanced stage of his diabetes. This employee had two grown children of his own, one who was starting graduate school and the other finishing a senior year in high school. I suspected that deep down the employee was concerned about his own children's fates if he himself ended up following in the medical steps of his father. While I had nothing to offer that day but a sympathetic ear, his story inspired me to become someone who would have something to give such employees. I am now in a position to give him, his coworkers, and his employer the knowledge of a workplace alternative to the status quo of chronic disease. I now know that most chronic diseases, including diabetes, can be prevented and even reversed through workplace lifestyle changes. Some may think that creating a plant-based workplace is an insurmountable, unrealistic task, but ultimately it is something that can be achieved through initiating a ripple effect. Helping that one employee is the first step to transforming not only the entire workplace food environment, but also the families and communities that environment sustains.

2 | OBESITY

Definition

Most workplace food environments reflect the community in which they are based. New Zealand public health expert Boyd Swinburn is credited with coining the term "obesogenic environment," defined as the sum of influences the surroundings, opportunities, or conditions of life have on promoting obesity in individuals or populations.[12] In other words, the term obesogenic is a way to describe an environment that encourages or promotes weight gain and obesity by surrounding individuals with a plethora of unhealthy, calorically-dense convenience foods and that discourages physical activity. It was during Swinburn's 1980s obesity and diabetes studies on Arizona's Pima Indian Reservation that he came to understand the role the environment plays in chronic disease: "Driving down to the reservation from Phoenix, I realized that it was not things within the body that were determining the health problems of this population. I came to the conclusion that obviously the driver of diabetes was obesity and that obesity was just a normal physiological response to an abnormal environment."[13]

The plight of the Pima Indians has been illuminating for epidemiologists and public health researchers. Ethnobotany sheds additional light on changes in the Pima diet over time. The ancestors of the Pima Indians settled the Gila River Valley in what later came to colonial era Mexico.[14] Over the years, the Pima Indians adapted to desert life by creating an intricate system of irrigation channels to support cultivation of corn, beans, and squash – all healthy plant-based foods.[14] In the mid-1800s, the United States purchased a section of northern Mexico, which became modern Arizona and New Mexico, under the Gadsden Purchase.[14, 15] This allowed the United States to establish railroads connecting the east and west coasts.[15] The influx of white settlers at the turn of the century led to the eventual diversion of the water supply that supported the Pima agricultural system.[14]

The forced change to Pima farming practices would have significant consequences for their food intake and physical activity levels for generations to come. Their lifestyles changed from a physically vigorous agricultural production economy to one of famine and physical inactivity.[14] Their lifestyle rapidly shifted from a low-fat, high-complex carbohydrate diet and regular physical activity to a sedentary lifestyle fed on a diet consisting of over 40% fat, mostly from animals and processed convenience foods.[14, 16] The timing of these lifestyle and environmental changes correlates with a rise in documented Pima diabetes cases.[14] In 1900, only one case of diabetes was recorded; in 1937, twenty-one cases were recorded. By the 1950s, the prevalence of diabetes increased tenfold, and by 1965 the Pima set a tragic record with the highest diabetes prevalence ever documented in the United States.[14]

Obesity is a disease characterized by accumulation of excessive body fat. Evolutionarily speaking, fat reserves served as a survival mechanism during periods of starvation, such that people with more body fat survived better during times of famine than did leaner people. In this way, nature has selectively bred humans over countless generations to rapidly accumulate fat. Thus, although some may think obesity is a choice, this chronic condition is far more complex than mere personal choice and is in fact considered a disease with numerous contributing environmental factors, including diet, physical activity level, and even stress. Specifically, there are genetic factors that predispose some people to weight gain and obesity. Obesity can influence normal body function and decrease life expectancy.[17] Furthermore, the American Medical Association, the Food and Drug Administration, the National Institutes of Health, and even the Internal Revenue Service all recognize obesity as a disease.[17]

Obesity is determined by assessing an individual's body mass index (BMI), the measure of a person's weight measured in kilograms (kg) relative to height measured in meters squared (m²):

$$BMI = \frac{Weight\ (kg)}{Height\ (m^2)}$$

The United States Centers for Disease Control and Prevention (CDC) designates BMI categories as shown in Table 2.0 [18]:

Table 2.0 - BMI weight classifications for adults [18]

BMI	Weight Classification
<18.5	Underweight
18.5 to 24.9	Normal
25 to 29.9	Overweight
30 to 34.9	Obese – Class 1
35 to 39.9	Obese – Class 2
40 and above	Obese – Class 3
	Also referred to as "severe" or "extreme" obesity

BMI is not a perfect measure because it does not consider body composition, meaning it does not take into account lean body mass relative to fat mass. A body builder could have a deceptively high BMI due to high lean body muscle mass with a relatively low percent body fat. Conversely, a person with low lean body mass and high fat mass could be considered healthy based on BMI alone. Despite these flaws, BMI can serve as a preliminary assessment tool, and is currently the globally accepted approach to measuring obesity.

Beyond merely measuring obesity, studies also show the importance of considering where on a person's body fat resides. Individuals with higher levels of abdominal body fat (or visceral fat) are at higher risk for diabetes, coronary heart disease, among others. This excessive belly fat is popularly described as the "apple" shape. However, people with higher levels of fat below the waistline, namely the hip and thigh areas, or "pear" shape, are at less risk. Thus, if there are two people with the same BMI, the person with the "apple" shape is at higher risk than the person with a "pear" shape. The World Health Organization considers the waist circumference measurement cutoff points of >95 cm (37.4 inches) for men and >80 cm (31.5 inches) for women to be associated with obesity and greater risk of chronic disease.[19]

In lieu of using a more accurate magnetic resonance imaging (MRI) or dual energy x-ray absorptiometry (DEXA) scan, which are typically found in academic research settings to measure body composition, the waist-to-hip ratio (WHR) or waist-to-height ratio (WHrT) may be more practical for assessing body fat distribution.[20, 21] WHR and WHrT are calculated using either inches (in) or centimeters (cm) in the following manner:

$$WHR = \frac{Waist\ circumference\ (in\ or\ cm)}{Hip\ circumference\ (in\ or\ cm)}$$

$$WHrT = \frac{Waist\ circumference\ (in\ or\ cm)}{Height\ (in\ or\ cm)}$$

Although there is no official consensus among the World Health Organization and CDC on healthy targets for WHR or WHrT, the literature suggests that a WHR of >0.8 for women and >0.9 for men, and a WHrT of ≥0.54 for both sexes, are associated with obesity.[22, 23]

Prevalence and Economic Impact

Obesity is a significant workplace and broader societal issue. Both the news media and scholarly publications have discussed ad nauseam the way obesity levels have drastically increased over the last several decades among all American age and gender populations. The World Health Organization estimates that 2.8 million people die prematurely each year due to obesity.[24] That works out to the same annual fatality rates as five Titanic ships sinking or 15 fully loaded jumbo jets crashing daily. In 2014 the McKinsey Global Institute – the research arm of the global management consulting firm McKinsey & Company – reported that the worldwide economic burden of obesity is $2.0 trillion a year, or 2.8% of the global GDP (Gross Domestic Product), and that its economic impact is equivalent to that of smoking, war, and terrorism.[25]

The prevalence of American adults with obesity was 13% in 1960-1962 and held somewhat steady until the late 1980s to early 1990s, when it jumped to 23% 1988-1994, with continued rise to almost 40% by 2015-2016.[26]   Figure 2.0 illustrates the trend since 1999.

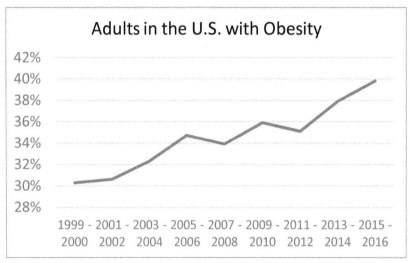

Figure 2.0: Adult obesity trends in the United States[26]

Adult obesity in the workplace has devastating impacts on the children adult employees support.   Obesity levels in American children has tripled since 1980. In comparison to adult obesity trends, childhood obesity grew from 13.9% in 1999 to 17.2% in 2014, and was estimated at 18.3% in 2017.[27, 28] Research clearly shows that children with obesity are more likely to become adults with obesity; and that children with two parents suffering from obesity are 10 to 12 times more likely to have obesity themselves.[29, 30] In addition, children with obesity have higher healthcare costs due to more outpatient appointments, emergency room visits, and drug prescriptions.[31] Furthermore, children with obesity are more likely to suffer from low self-esteem, social isolation, depression, and discrimination.[32] These problems can lead to poor academic performance. In fact, one large study found that children with obesity were not only more likely to have health problems, but also experienced an increase in school absences (missing 10 or more days), more course failures, and reduced interest in school subjects compared to children of a healthy weight.[33] These children of companies' adult employees are often dependents on employer healthcare plans as well as the next generation of talent that business leaders will want to recruit. It is therefore prudent for all stakeholders, including the private sector business community, to make it a priority to take preventative measures that address this obesity epidemic.

Obesity is not a uniquely American problem. Globally, 10% of men and 14% of women had obesity in 2008, compared to 5% for men and 8% for women in 1980.[34] The increase is mainly seen in countries with higher income levels, as well as those that have adopted the "Western" style of eating and consumption of ultra-processed foods as is the case of people living in the Oceania region and Polynesian Islands. Figure 2.1 depicts the average change in BMI from 1980 to 2008 among various regions around the globe for both males and females.[34]

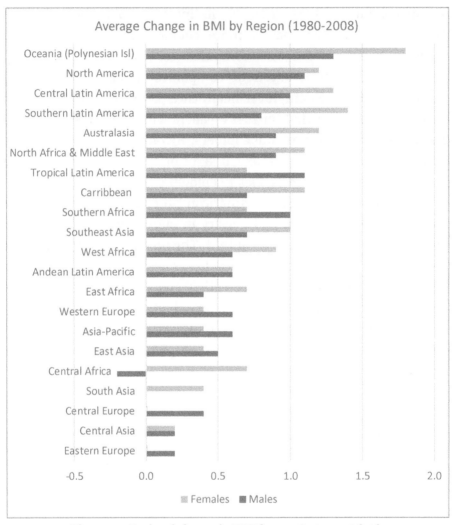

Figure 2.1: Regional change in BMI from 1980 to 2008 [34]

Contributing Factors

Obesity is considered a complex, multi-factorial disease. Beyond the mere mathematical relationship between calorie intake and calories burned, there are several contributing genetic and hormonal factors at play, as well as environmental and lifestyle influences, such as food type, physical inactivity, and psychological stress. Figure 2.2 illustrates the complex causes of obesity.

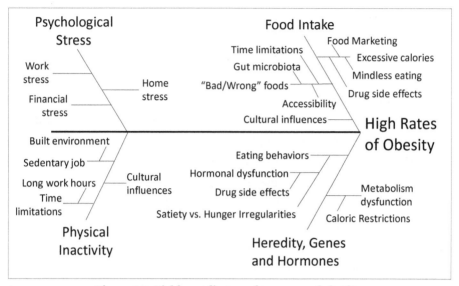

Figure 2.2: Fishbone diagram for causes of obesity

Heredity, Genes, and Hormones

Popular discussions of obesity rarely cover genetic causes. Before we discuss the role of genetics in obesity, let us explore the key hormones that interact with the brain and other organs in the body to regulate appetite, food intake, and body weight. Hormones control hunger, satiation (or fullness), and fat development. If these hormones control whether we want to eat, then having a workplace food environment loaded with calorically-dense foods high in saturated fat, dietary cholesterol, sugar, and salt sets employees up for health dangers. This is especially true for employees who may have a hormone dysfunction.

Under normal conditions, when the stomach is empty, the body releases a hormone that stimulates appetite. After a meal, neural signals to the brain decrease appetite and food intake with the release of different hormones, and the appetite stimulation hormone dissipates after a meal. As blood glucose rises after eating, insulin and other hormones are released, further decreasing appetite and food consumption.

Humans have somewhere between 19,000 and 20,000 genes.[35] Scientists do not yet fully understand how these genes interact. However, research reveals more every day about the interaction between genes, as well as between genes and the environment. The study of the interaction between an individual's genes and the environment is known as epigenetics, which aims to characterize how the environment induces chemical changes that determine whether genes are expressed. Since there are several genes involved in facilitating the release of appetite and body weight regulation hormones, any replication errors, loss of function, or mutations in these genes could predispose a person to weight gain.

For example, one human gene provides instructions for making the hormone leptin, which regulates body weight. This hormone is made from the body's fat cells. As fat stores increase, leptin production also increases. Leptin binds to receptors in the brain that control hunger and, under normal conditions, tells the brain that the individual is full. However, common gene mutations can cause dysfunction in leptin signaling, leading to excessive hunger and weight gain when the individual does not experience a feeling of satiety.

Another gene is responsible for making and regulating the ghrelin hormone that stimulates appetite.[36] Ghrelin is released by the stomach when the stomach is empty. It is a powerful appetite stimulant that acts on the hypothalamus of the brain to secrete growth hormone, and gene mutations can promote obesity.[36] The hormone obestatin is thought to have an appetite-decreasing effect, resulting in a reduction of food intake.[36]

Existing studies are inconclusive, but it is possible that a gene mutation could disrupt this obestatin hormone appetite-decreasing function, leading to overeating and weight gain.

Here is worth introducing the notion of set-point theory. The set-point theory proposes that body weight is metabolically preprogrammed into an individual, typically based on the genes with which they were born. Proponents of this theory cite cases of patients who undergo gastric banding, a surgical procedure that involves implanting a mechanical restriction (band) to reduce stomach capacity and caloric intake, and who eventually regain weight despite the procedure. Similarly, a person adopting a calorically restricted diet – eating 500, 700 or 1,000 fewer calories each day – will also regain weight. Published research data support that weight is regained over time with these types of caloric restrictions.[37] However, the shortcoming of the set-point theory is that the effects observed are confounded by the role of our obesogenic community and workplace environments. Therefore, people with a predisposition to excessive weight or obesity may find success in "fighting the trajectory"[17] with specific lifestyle changes related to food intake type, physical activity, and psychological stress management, all of which have strong environmental influences, and all of which are potential components of a workplace environment.

Food Intake

Obesity has typically been perceived as a mathematically simplistic caloric input-output issue, or as what health experts call "overnutrition" or a "positive energy balance" over time, meaning caloric (energy) intake exceeds caloric (energy) expenditure. For example, having a consistent positive energy balance of even just 50 calories per day (equivalent to a quarter of a candy bar, or a one-third of a 12-ounce can of soda) translates to a weight gain of 26 pounds over five years. This phenomenon is known as creeping obesity. Daily energy expenditure comprises three elements:

1. Basal energy expenditure is the energy required for the body's resting metabolism. This is the energy it takes to support the body's tissues and daily functions.
2. Thermal food effect is the energy required to absorb, store, and metabolize food.
3. Physical activity energy expenditure is any form of muscular activity, such as daily body motion and exercise. This can vary greatly in the workplace environment depending on physical workplace design.

Because of the responsive nature of our metabolism's evolutionary design, calorie reduction diets cause our basal energy expenditure and thermal food effect to also decrease. For our ancestors, this was a survival mechanism during periods of food scarcity, but it is not so helpful to us today. Furthermore, as fewer calories are consumed, there is less energy for physical activity because the body seeks to maintain homeostasis by reducing energy expenditure. Therefore, calorie restriction alone is not an effective way to lose weight over time. The latest research supports focusing instead on the type of food consumed coupled with daily physical activity as a more effective way to lose weight and keep it off.

Foods known to spike insulin are prime culprits in obesity trends. High intakes of ultra-processed foods cause insulin levels to surge, promoting weight gain and obesity. Ultra-processed foods are typically high in salt, sugar, and saturated fat, and include sweet or savory snacks, soft drinks, ready-to-eat meals, and other industrial formulations manufactured with often unpronounceable additive ingredients developed by food chemists to change food color, texture, and taste, appealing to human taste buds and prolonging shelf life. American households take in an estimated

60% of their daily caloric intake from ultra-processed foods, and diets high in ultra-processed foods are associated with reductions or even deficiencies in essential dietary components, such as protein, fiber, and vitamins.[38, 39] The ultra-processed food intake for other "Western" countries is not much different: Canada, 55%; United Kingdom, 51%; and Norway, 49%.[39] Following this trend, Brazil, Chile, and other Latin American countries have experienced dramatic increases in obesity and diabetes cases in recent decades, which public health officials attribute to the influx of ultra-processed foods.[40-43]

The average US intake of added sugars amounts to almost 300 calories per day, mostly in the form of ultra-processed foods.[44] These foods are desirable because they are inexpensive, convenient, and designed by food chemists to be highly palatable and even addictive.[45] These ultra-processed foods are often calorically dense, but not nutrient dense. Unsurprisingly, studies have found statistically significant associations between ultra-processed food consumption and obesity levels.[41, 46-48] These ultra-processed foods usually comprise the majority of food products sold in workplace vending machines and cafeterias.

One mechanism through which processed foods encourage obesity lies in the symbiotic relationship between humans and their intestinal microorganisms. Researchers have learned a great deal in recent decades about how gut microbiota – the community of microorganisms that make up the intestinal microbiome – influences human physiological responses to hormones and metabolism. While this area of study is still relatively new, there is strong research evidence that physiological responses from the gut microbiome may determine susceptibility to weight gain. Specifically, *Bacteroidetes* and *Firmicutes* bacteria have been of interest as these are the dominant microbes in the gut microbiome of Western populations.[49] Individuals with obesity have a higher ratio of *Firmicutes* to *Bacteroidetes* than people of healthy weight.[49] Excessive quantities of *Firmicutes* have been associated with weight gain, and are believed to promote this trend because they metabolize intestinal food matter more efficiently.[50] Indeed, since diet is the main driver of gut microbiome species composition, the types of foods an individual eats may be more important than originally thought.

Gut microbes from the healthier *Bacteroidetes* family are more prominent in individuals whose diets are rich in complex plant fibers, the fermentation of which produces beneficial short chain fatty acids in the intestines.[51, 52] Short chain fatty acid production appears to play an important role in appetite regulation, thus preventing weight gain. Fiber-rich foods are those derived from whole plant foods (i.e., vegetables, fruits, whole grains, legumes) with minimal processing, whereas animal products have no fiber and ultra-processed foods have little, if any, fiber.

In summary, we know that insulin and other hormones can promote weight gain when production is improperly stimulated. We know that the gut microbiome in people with obesity is different from people of healthy weight, and that the relative abundance of beneficial *Bacteroidetes* bacteria is associated with diets rich in complex plant fiber. Imagine if every business moved towards a workplace food environment model based on foods that help employees achieve and maintain a healthy body weight!

Role of Environmental Queues

After years of corporate wellness program models that promote monotonous selections of "some healthy choices" in workplace food venues, but that still maintain an ample supply of dopamine-triggering unhealthy foods (i.e., repeated exposure to foods that activate the neurotransmitter, dopamine affecting sensations of pleasurable rewards and junk food addictive behaviors), it's not surprising that companies continue to see their bottom lines hit hard by healthcare costs. In my personal workplace experiences, healthy cafeteria choices often meant lame salad saucers of iceberg lettuce with desiccated grated carrot and a piece of mushy tomato, or the wilted brown banana that sat neglected and lonely in a wicker bowl for a fruit. Most workplace food environments don't make it easy for people to eat healthy, especially with the sort of job pressures from deadlines, understaffing, and ever-increasing performance expectations that encourage eating for speed and convenience. Depending on the thoughtfulness of planning, the workplace food environment can facilitate the kinds of human gene expression or suppression that either contribute to health or disease promotion. This is an opportunity for companies to be part of the solution by making it easier for employees to prevent or reverse obesity and other chronic diseases. I will discuss the business case for doing so in a later section, but for now let's cover a few key points that contribute to food intake "choices."

Mindless eating is defined in Brian Wansink's book of the same name as eating food without paying adequate attention to what and how much is being eaten.[53] Food psychology practices are frequently used both to help people make healthier choices and to market food products. For example, Dr. Brad Appelhans of Chicago's Rush University introduced campus vending machines that imposed a 25-second countdown delay when dispensing unhealthy snacks to give consumers more time to think about the purchase and perhaps change their choice.[54] These vending machines, aptly called "Delays to Influence Snack Choice," were installed all over campus, and after several weeks brought about a 5% increase in the proportion of healthy snack sales.[54]

The emphasis on "value," or getting more for less, exacerbates mindless eating, resulting in excessive food intake and subsequent weight gain. Unless the consumer is mindful, there is a high likelihood of unwitting overconsumption. I have certainly experienced this myself. For example, I remember stopping at a gas station in rural Louisiana after a bicycle race to fill up my gas tank before my 3-hour drive home. It was a typical hot, humid summer day. I had mixed nuts in the car for snacking and wanted an ice-cold Coke, something I only consumed during long, intense training rides or after races. There was a stack of Styrofoam cups lining the stand where the soft drink dispensers were located, with three possible sizes advertised in large bold font: 16, 24, and 48 ounces, and all for the same price, $1.49. I chose the smallest size possible. Even though I was mindful to grab the cup size I truly wanted, I still had a nagging sensation that I had overpaid and could have gotten more for the same amount of money.

Researchers at the University of Pennsylvania use the term "unit bias" to describe the phenomenon exemplified by my Coke buying experience, and have found that portion sizes indisputably influence how much a person consumes.[55] This is thought in part to be due to perceived pressures to finish a serving regardless of satiety or fullness.[55] Their study looked at the consumption of free snacks (i.e., soft pretzels, Tootsie Rolls, and M&Ms) offered on a public counter in an office building and a large apartment building in Philadelphia.[55] They varied the sizes of the unit portions either by changing the size of the snack or the utensil used to dish it up, and found that in all cases on the days where the unit sizes were larger, substantially more of the snack was taken.[55] This perceived pressure to get the most one can in a serving, and to finish the portion completely reminds me of growing up where my friend's mom encouraged us at dinner to get accepted into "the clean plate club," because finishing the portion served on the plate was behavior to be rewarded.

Regardless of BMI, most people are unaware of how their food environment influences their daily dietary decisions. A 2008 study demonstrates that people are either unable or unwilling to report external factors that influence their eating behavior, including reasons for starting or finishing a meal, as well as how much is consumed during the meal.[56] Most people are unaware that they are influenced by how much other people around them are eating, but will "generate several alternative explanations for their behavior... rooted in common-sense theories," such as being hungry or full.[56] The study concludes that if people are not aware or are unwilling to acknowledge external environmental queues shaping food consumption, expecting them to follow healthy dietary patterns is unrealistic[56]. I would go a step further and say that it is near impossible in the current workplace food environment. In a 2015 study, researchers looked at added sugar intake and BMI, and found a sizable discrepancy between self-reported intake versus what urine samples showed.[57] Specifically, analyzing urine sample data revealed a positive correlation between sugar intake and BMI (high BMI associated with high sugar intake), whereas self-reported data showed an inverse relationship (high BMI associated with reported lower sugar intake), suggesting people with higher BMIs may be unaware or unwilling to acknowledge how much sugar they actually consume.[57]

I think many of us, if we are honest with ourselves, can identify moments in our own lives in which we have experienced how the workplace food environment promotes mindless eating. I can't count the occasions when I used to stop by a coworker's desk just to grab a piece of candy from her conveniently placed bowl, or swing by the vending machine before a conference call to snack on something crunchy because I was stressed about the topic of the meeting. I wasn't eating these things because I was hungry; it was simply because they were there. Imagine how a more thoughtfully designed workplace food environment could address employees' mindless eating, perhaps by ensuring that healthy foods are the only ones available for free or in easy reach!

Physical Activity and Psychological Stress

Two other factors contributing to obesity are physical inactivity and psychological stress. These topics are vast and worthy of their own texts, but they are essential to mention here given their relevance to workplace conditions that contribute to obesity.

In both the workplace and our broader communities, the need for physical activity has been reduced due to technological advances. Daily physical activity is an important way not only to reduce weight but also to keep it off.[58]   For those with a metabolic program or predisposition for obesity, regular exercise is proven to help "fight the trajectory" of set-point weight gain.[17] Physical activity can take the form of scheduled exercise or can be directly integrated into regular daily activities. As a personal anecdote, I first experienced the ability to fight the trajectory of what could have been my set-point weight gain during my senior year in college with physical activity from my part-time job. For example, looking at this 1994 photo of my parents and me (center) taken on my university graduation day would lead many to believe my body weight could potentially be metabolically programed, as described by the set-point theory earlier, to have obesity (Figure 2.3), but in the photo I do not exhibit excessive weight or obesity.

However, the reader should know that I was about 20 pounds heavier my junior year, and at the beginning of my senior year I moved out of my parents' home into my very own "Laverne and Shirley" apartment where I also worked as the building janitor in exchange for reduced rent. Janitorial duties in this 20-suite apartment complex involved climbing four stories multiple times a week to carry trash to the garage, and then from the garage out to the curb on trash day. I was also responsible for vacuuming the carpet in public areas, as well as for sweeping and mopping the tiled floors of the back entrances and laundry room. My physical activity from life tasks alone increased substantially compared to when I had lived at home, and while I did not consciously try to lose weight, the changes in my environment naturally took the pounds off. Dan Buettner, author of *The Blue Zone Solutions*, might describe this as my environment "nudging" me into healthy behaviors of physical activity.

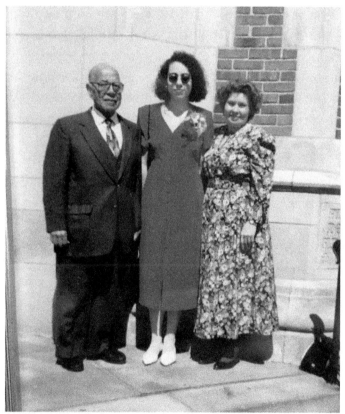

Figure 2.3: Dad, me, and Mom at my college graduation, John Carroll University (Ohio), May 1994.

In addition to obesity, the World Health Organization estimates that physical inactivity contributes to 30% of heart disease cases, 27% of type 2 diabetes cases, and 21-25% of breast and colon cancer cases.[59]   It recommends that adults get at least 150 minutes of moderate – or 75 minutes of vigorous – physical activity each week, but more than these recommended minimums is certainly better.[59] For many people, that could work out to 30 minutes or more of moderate physical activity daily. For those with obesity, starting an exercise program typically requires guidance from a physician. Short bouts of walking are commonly prescribed in the beginning with gradual increases to duration and intensity. For a person with a history of obesity, many experts advise getting 300 minutes per week or 60 minutes per day to maintain weight loss over the course of his or her lifetime.[58]   And even if the individual struggles with weight loss, losing even 5% of body weight can have meaningful metabolic benefits for a person with obesity.

Chronic psychological stresses at work and home may also contribute to obesity through physiological responses to "stress eating" of junk foods. Studies show a positive association between psychological stress and a diet high in sugar and fat.[60, 61] These dietary and physiological responses to stress can be exacerbated by the body's own stress hormones, such as cortisol. Cortisol is secreted by the adrenal gland and helps convert protein building blocks to the simple sugar glucose. This was evolutionarily useful for fueling "fight or flight" events for survival, providing the individual with a sudden adrenalin boost and subsequently stimulating muscles to take action. Today, however, we are unlikely to be chased by a predatory animal. The elevated cortisol levels from chronic psychological or emotional stress that may have once helped our ancestors survive puts us at increased risk for weight gain. Furthermore,   increased   cortisol   levels   from   chronic psychological stress are proven to increase blood glucose levels, resulting in abdominal fat accumulation and insulin resistance, both of which are precursors to type 2 diabetes.[62]

Obesity Linked to Other Diseases and Conditions

A vast quantity of studies have shown strong associations between obesity and other disease conditions, increasing the risk of premature death.[58, 63] It is estimated that people with obesity lose between 3 and 10 years of life compared to people without obesity.[63] The quality of life for people with obesity is lower due to pain from musculoskeletal conditions, mobility issues, social stigma, negative stereotypes, discrimination,[64] as well as increased likelihood of acquiring one or more chronic diseases, also referred to as a "comorbidity."[63] One large pooled study found that people with severe (Class III) obesity experience a life expectancy reduction similar to that of smokers.[65] In addition to reduced life expectancy, these comorbidities are costly and lower quality of life, because they involve more frequent visits to medical clinics, as well as long-term dependence on prescription medications and the adverse side effects of continual use of these drugs. The following is a list of comorbidities linked to obesity:

- Type 2 Diabetes
- Hypertension
- Dyslipidemia
- Atherosclerosis
- Heart Disease
- Stroke
- Cancer
- Sleep Apnea
- Osteoarthritis
- Liver Disease
- Gallbladder Disease

- Reproductive Complications

The next two chapters will dive deeper into the chronic diseases for which obesity is a contributing factor; specifically, type 2 diabetes, as well as cardiovascular and cerebrovascular diseases.

3 | TYPE 2 DIABETES

Definition

Under normal conditions, when a person eats a peanut butter and jelly sandwich, the carbohydrates are broken down into glucose. As the glucose is absorbed through cells lining the digestive tract, blood glucose level rises. In response to the rise in blood glucose, cells in the pancreas are stimulated to release the hormone insulin into the blood stream. The insulin signals to the body's cells that it is time to take up glucose from the blood stream. The glucose then provides energy for functions like muscle contraction. The term "insulin resistance" describes a medical condition in which the cells no longer respond to this signal, such that glucose is not taken up and increases to problematic levels in the bloodstream. Conversely, when an individual has "high insulin sensitivity," it means the pancreas is working well and insulin is successfully signaling to cells to take up glucose.

The main characteristic of diabetes is hyperglycemia (excessively high blood sugar) resulting from defects in how the body produces insulin, how insulin functions, or both. Dysfunctional insulin metabolism is at play in what is commonly known as diabetes. Diabetes mellitus, the formal term, is not a single disease, but a group of endocrine disorders that vary in origin and severity. There are four classifications of diabetes mellitus: type 1, type 2, gestational, and diabetes caused by other conditions. Type 2 diabetes comprises most of all diabetes cases in the United States and globally. Table 3.0 further describes the classification of each diabetes type.

The signs and symptoms associated with type 2 diabetes are insidious and initially undetectable, but tend to progress over time. More advanced signs and symptoms of type 2 diabetes include: increased thirst, frequent urination, increased hunger, feeling tired, blurred vision, tingling in the feet or hands, sores that do not heal, and unexplained weight loss.[66] In addition to common signs and symptoms, type 2 diabetes is diagnosed based on blood tests. Two common blood test threshold values used to diagnose a person with type 2 diabetes are Hemoglobin A_{1c} ≥6.5%, and fasting plasma glucose ≥126 mg/dL (70 to 100 mg/dL is considered normal).

Table 3.0: Summary of types of diabetes [67, 68]

Classification	Description
Type 1 Diabetes Mellitus	Autoimmune condition resulting in a lack of insulin due to beta cell destruction; requires insulin injections to manage blood glucose levels in normal range.
	Risk is linked to specific gene associations, but also has an environmental component that has not definitively been determined.
	Commonly diagnosed in children and young adults. Historically, referred to as "juvenille diabetes."
Type 2 Diabetes Mellitus	Combination of abnormal insulin secretion from the pancreas, and insulin resistance of the body's cells to insulin signaling.
	Risks associated with excessive weight, obesity, physical inactivity, poor nutrition, and family history.
	Historically referred to as "adult onset" diabetes, but due to the increased prevalence among children and adolescents, is now referred to as "type 2 diabetes" and comprises 90-95% of all diabetes cases in the United States.
Gestational Diabetes Mellitus [66, 67]	Diabetes during pregnancy where the body is not able to produce enough insulin or utilize the insulin.
	It is associated with increased risk of type 2 diabetes for both mother and child, where excessive weight (fat mass) and certain genes play a role in the onset of this type of diabetes.
	Women who are overweight or obese at the time of pregnancy are at a greater risk of a gestational diabetes diagnosis.
Diabetes due to other causes	Diabetes brought on by other conditions, such as Cystic fibrosis or drug (chemical) induction.

Prevalence and Economic Impact

Diabetes is one of the most significant public health concerns globally in terms of both prevalence and costs. There were 422 million people living with diabetes in 2014 worldwide.[69] In 2015, an estimated 30.3 million people in the United States had diabetes, of which an estimated 7.4 million were considered undiagnosed.[70] The global economic burden of diabetes was estimated at $1.3 trillion in 2015.[71] In 2012, economic costs of diabetes in the United States reached $245 billion, of which $176 billion comprises direct medical costs and the remaining $69 billion was due to lost productivity.[72] The American economic costs for 2012 increase to $322 billion when factoring in prediabetes.[72]

In 1935, the prevalence of diabetes in the United States was 0.37%; in 1960, 0.91%; in 1980, 3.7%; and by 2015 rates grew to 8.7% of the population.[70, 73] Figure 3.0 illustrates the annual trend in the United States since 1980.[74] This trend coincides with the increase in obesity prevalence.

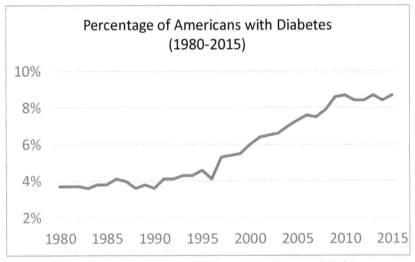

Figure 3.0: Historical trend of Americans with diagnosed diabetes [74]

Contributing Factors

The primary contributing factors to type 2 diabetes are excessive weight, obesity, and physical inactivity. The Obesity Society, a nonprofit industry group comprises healthcare professionals and academic experts, estimates that almost 90% of people with type 2 diabetes have excessive weight or obesity.[75] The chances of getting type 2 diabetes increases with age, explaining why it used to be called adult onset diabetes, but due to a growing childhood obesity epidemic, children and adolescents are being diagnosed with this disease condition more frequently. Another risk factor is pregnancy, in the case of gestational diabetes, where there is an increased future risk of both mother and child acquiring type 2 diabetes. One study found that children born after the mother was diagnosed with diabetes had almost a fourfold increased risk of suffering from diabetes and obesity compared to children born before maternal diabetes diagnosis, suggesting that disease exposure, and not heredity, is the cause.[76]

The lifestyle factors contributing to type 2 diabetes are largely poor diet and physical inactivity. Diets high in ultra-processed packaged convenience foods (including refined sugars and grains) as well as diets rich in processed meats, cheeses, and other animal products, promote this disease risk. This fiber-deficient Western dietary pattern is low in vegetables, fruits, whole grains, and legumes. Furthermore, the risk of type 2 diabetes also increases with a sedentary lifestyle. One study shows that walking briskly over 20 minutes each day (or ≥ 2.5 hours per week) reduces the risk of type 2 diabetes by 30% compared to very little walking.[77]

Type 2 diabetes can promote the onset of other chronic diseases. In fact, type 2 diabetes is among the leading causes of blindness, limb amputation, heart disease and stroke. When type 2 diabetes progresses unmonitored for a long period of time, it can advance to cause chronic kidney disease or renal failure. When this happens, the damage is considered permanent and the patient must go on dialysis. Kidneys are the body's filtration system removing excessive wastes and fluids from the body. Dialysis is an artificial kidney replacement procedure that uses equipment and devices to filter and remove excessive by-products of metabolism from the blood. Dialysis is extremely disruptive to an individual's life, because it either involves multiple trips to a dialysis treatment center each week, or having a catheter surgically placed within the abdomen and undergoing dialysis at home four times per day including during sleep at night.

A 2015 U.S. Renal Data System report notes that there has been a "47-fold increase in dialysis over the last 40 years because of the increase in diabetes, hypertension and other chronic diseases."[78] Despite the exponential growth rates in the dialysis industry (along with healthcare costs associated with it), the good news is that this disease is largely preventable. People with prediabetes or early stages of type 2 diabetes can either halt the progression of this disease, or in many cases, even reverse it through a meaningful change in diet and regular physical activity, thus avoiding the dismal need to even consider a future at the mercy of renal dialysis. The question for business leaders is this: Is your company's workplace food environment helping to promote or prevent type 2 diabetes? If the foods offered are ultra-processed; calorically dense; and high in saturated fat, sugar and salt, the workplace itself may be promoting this disease.

4 | CARDIOVASCULAR AND CEREBROVASCULAR DISEASES

Definition

The primary purpose of the cardiovascular system is to ensure that oxygenated blood and nutrients flow to organs and tissues, and that waste products from cellular metabolism are removed. This system is also responsible for hormone transport, as well as regulation of body temperature, pH balance, and other physiological processes. Diseases of the cardiovascular system adversely impact the system's ability to carry out all of these normal functions. The focus of this next part will be on the other major sub-conditions of the cardiovascular and cerebrovascular, or heart and brain circulatory, systems. Specifically, hypertension, dyslipidemia, atherosclerosis, stroke and aneurysm.

Hypertension or "high blood pressure" occurs when the force of the blood against the arterial walls is too high. This condition is also referred to as the "silent killer" because people experience no noticeable symptoms and do not suspect they have hypertension unless they happen to have a routine physical exam during which their blood pressure is assessed. Blood pressure is measured in millimeters of mercury or "mmHg" for short. In 2017, a task force that included the American College of Cardiology and the American Heart Association published new clinical practice guidelines that lowered the threshold for what is considered "hypertension" from ≥140 mmHg systolic or ≥90 mmHg diastolic to ≥130 mmHg systolic or ≥80 mmHg diastolic.[79] As a consequence of this threshold change, the estimated number of people in the United States with hypertension increased from 29% to 46%.[79, 80] The task force chose to adjust the threshold based on medical complications observed in clinical settings at even these lower blood pressure levels. Changing the criteria for diagnosing hypertension would necessitate earlier intervention, before hypertension is able to escalate to a serious event or disease condition, such as myocardial infarction (heart attack) or stroke.[79] Table 4.0 provides an overview of the different blood pressure classifications from the American Heart Association.[81]

Table 4.0: American Heart Association blood pressure classifications[81]

Classification	Systolic (mmHg)		Diastolic (mmHg)
Normal	<120	and	<80
Elevated	120-129	and	<80
Hypertension Stage 1	130-139	or	80-89
Hypertension Stage 2	≥140	or	≥90
Hypertensive Crisis *Seek immediate medical attention*	>180	and/or	>120

Systolic measurements represent the ventricular contraction phase, while diastolic measurements represent ventricular relaxation.

The pulse pressure is the difference between systolic and diastolic blood pressure (i.e., systolic minus diastolic) and may be an indicator of damaged blood vessels and increased cardiac risk. Elevated pulse pressure (≥60) can be due to a stiffening of the aorta due to plaque (or fatty deposits) on the arterial walls.

Dyslipidemia occurs when blood cholesterol and triglyceride levels are at unhealthy levels. Cholesterol is a biomarker used to assess an individual's risk of cardiovascular and cerebrovascular diseases. Elevated or low cholesterol levels can be genetic but are also influenced by lifestyle (diet and physical activity). Cholesterol is a form of lipid (fat) that has a waxy texture and is found in our blood. Our bodies naturally make cholesterol, which is an important precursor for the synthesis of steroid hormones and the bile acids we need for digestion and absorption of lipids in the intestines. However, when too much cholesterol, specifically LDL cholesterol, is stored in the blood it can wreak havoc on the cardiovascular and cerebrovascular system over time. LDL (low density lipoprotein) or "bad" cholesterol can oxidize and eventually form plaque in the arterial wall. That plaque builds up and blocks blood flow, thus causing a serious cardiovascular or cerebrovascular event. Insufficient HDL (high density lipoprotein), or "good" cholesterol, is also a risk factor. HDL cholesterol serves as a dump truck that removes harmful LDL cholesterol from the bloodstream, thus having higher HDL levels is considered beneficial. Low levels of HDL can be genetic; however, levels can also be low due to a sedentary lifestyle. It is worth mentioning that some studies involving a whole-food, plant-based diet intervention have shown reductions in HDL, however due to greater decreases in LDL the net effect is more protective. In addition, triglyceride levels, or the amount of fat in the blood, can also be a risk factor if levels are too high. Various factors such as excess body fat, physical inactivity, and smoking are associated with elevated triglyceride levels. To summarize, elevated LDL cholesterol and triglycerides, as well as with low levels of HDL cholesterol, are contributing factors to cardiovascular and cerebrovascular diseases. Table 4.1 details the different cholesterol level classifications.[82, 83]

Table 4.1: Cholesterol level categories[82, 83]

LDL "bad" cholesterol	<100 mg/dL	Optimal
	100-129 mg/dL	Near optimal
	130-159 mg/dL	Borderline high
	160-189 mg/dL	High
	≥190 mg/dL	Very high
HDL "good" cholesterol	<40 mg/dL	Major risk factor
	40-59 mg/dL	Normal
	≥60 mg/dL	Protective against heart disease
Triglycerides	<150 mg/dL	Normal
	150-199 mg/dL	Borderline high
	200-499 mg/dL	High
	≥500 mg/dL	Very high

Atherosclerosis involves injury to cells of the arterial walls when plaque accumulates over time, accompanied by an inflammatory response. Development of plaque occurs from consistently high levels of fat and cholesterol circulating in the bloodstream. The plaque forms along the walls of the arteries and impedes blood flow. The arterial walls then thicken and become less elastic. When the plaque becomes inflamed and ruptures, blood flow is significantly restricted, and depending on the location and the direction of flow, atherosclerosis will cause a heart attack, stroke, or peripheral artery disease (blockage in the leg). It is indisputable that heart disease and stroke are the leading causes of death in the United States and globally, which has a significant economic impact at multiple levels, across multiple sectors. The damage stems from the chronic pressure hypertension imposes on the arterial wall, as well as from oxidative damage caused by various unhealthy lifestyle habits, such as smoking, poor diet, and concomitant oxidized LDL cholesterol. Insulin resistance from type 2 diabetes is another contributing factor.

There are various types of strokes or aneurysm. Strokes can occur when the artery to the brain is blocked, inhibiting nutrients and oxygenated blood from reaching the brain and preventing carbon dioxide and waste from being removed. Such strokes can cause permanent damage to the brain or even death. Another type of stroke, often called a "mini stroke" (transient ischemic attack), is an early indicator of an impending, more serious stroke. When a mini-stroke occurs, the blockage is short-term and typically dissolves or dislodges within a few minutes. There is no long-term damage to the brain, but it is a strong warning sign and should not be disregarded. Hemorrhagic stroke is another type. It occurs when a blood vessel in the brain ruptures and the individual experiences bleeding in the brain. Rupture occurs when the blood vessel walls are weakened, usually due to hypertension. Hemorrhagic stroke is less common than other types, making up 15% of stroke cases.[84] However, it has the especially high mortality rate of 40%.[84] Related to the hemorrhagic stroke is the aneurysm. An aneurysm is the dilation and protruding, or "ballooning," of muscle at the point where cerebral arteries divide or split. Aneurysms develop with the presence of a constant flow of high blood pressure (hypertension), and are estimated to affect between 1.5-5% of the population.[85] If one or more aneurysms rupture, it becomes a hemorrhagic stroke.

Prevalence and Economic Impact

An alarming one in three adults have at least one type of cardiovascular or cerebrovascular disease. The leading cause of death in the United States and in other developed countries has been and continues to be heart disease. According to the Centers for Disease Control and Prevention, each year one in four deaths is due to heart disease.[86] Cardiovascular and cerebrovascular diseases cost the United States $320 billion per year in healthcare costs and lost productivity.[86] The amount of money spent on prescription drugs to prevent this number one killer in the United States is staggering. For example, statin (cholesterol lowering) drugs are a $17 billion per year industry in the United States, and because the growth in users is offset by the increased availability of generic options, this amount has held deceptively steady over the past decade.[87] Some believe that the amount spent on statin drugs is an inevitable price to pay for a reduction of cardiovascular events; however, I argue that companies wishing to reduce employee medical expenditures could achieve a double cost reduction benefit. Introducing a whole-food, plant-based diet into the workplace could reduce both statin prescriptions and cardiovascular procedures.

Up until the threshold changes in the clinical guidelines, the prevalence of hypertension held somewhat steady at around one third of the American adult population, with similar levels in both men and women. However, a breakdown of the data by race and age demographics showed higher rates for African Americans (42%) and people over age 60 (65%) compared to other races and younger age groups.[88] Existing studies are inconclusive as to why the prevalence of hypertension is disproportionately higher in the African American community, but some experts hypothesize that heredity and genetics; dietary patterns of foods high in salt, sugar, and fat; together with the environments that expose individuals to chronically high psychological stress may be culprits. These explanatory causes are common factors in many African American communities. Globally, the World Health Organization estimates the prevalence of hypertension to be around 40% based on the previous criteria (pre-2017 clinical practice guideline changes).[89] Countries with high per capita income levels have a lower hypertension prevalence at 35%, compared to countries with lower per capita incomes at just above 40%.[89] Globally, men exhibit slightly higher rates of hypertension than women; and regionally, Africa has the highest rates of hypertension at 46%.[89] The annual cost of hypertension in the United States and globally has been estimated to be $46 billion and $360 billion, respectively.[88, 90]

Contributing Factors

The risk factors for cardiovascular and cerebrovascular diseases are largely preventable, and are similar to those for diabetes. The American Heart Association has outlined seven indicators to assess when determining whether an individual is at high risk for cardiovascular or cerebrovascular diseases: blood pressure, cholesterol, blood glucose, physical activity level, diet, weight, and tobacco use. The American Heart Association (AHA) refers to these as "My Life Check – Life's Simple 7." The following information is based on the AHA's assessment guidelines:

1: Blood Pressure

Blood pressure at or over 130 mmHg systolic or over 80 mmHg diastolic is considered Stage 1 Hypertension and is a risk factor for cardiovascular and cerebrovascular diseases. The higher the blood pressure, the greater the risk. See Table 4.0 for the complete list of classifications for hypertension. Factors that contribute to an individual's risk for hypertension include: a poor diet of foods high in salt, fat, and sugar, but low in vegetables, fruits, whole grains and legumes; physical inactivity and sedentary lifestyle; tobacco use; excessive and chronic psychological stress; and excessive alcohol consumption.

In addition to these preventable risk factors, people with high cholesterol, obesity, and type 2 diabetes are often predisposed to hypertension.[79] Undiagnosed and untreated hypertension can strain the heart because it increases the workload required to pump blood through the body. Over time, this extra cardiac work can cause the muscle mass of the heart's left ventricle to grow disproportionately large, which can ultimately lead to heart failure. Hypertension can also increase the risk of kidney damage; in fact, it is the second leading cause of kidney failure after uncontrolled diabetes. This occurs because the kidneys are made up of tiny nephrons, which are like filtration tubes, that remove waste from the body's bloodstream. When arteries become blocked and damaged, so too do the nephrons in the kidneys. Kidney damage can then progress to the sort of chronic kidney disease that requires ongoing dialysis. Another risk associated with untreated hypertension is stroke. Hypertension can cause hemorrhagic stroke by weakening and rupturing blood vessels to the brain.

Combined complications of both hypertension and type 2 diabetes can also cause damage to eye tissues, resulting in vision impairment or loss. One study found between 47% to 69% increased risk of eye tissue damage in patients with hypertension, irrespective of being prescribed antihypertensive medications.[91]

2: Cholesterol

Elevated LDL ("bad") cholesterol and triglycerides, as well as with low levels of HDL ("good") cholesterol can contribute to cardiovascular and cerebrovascular disease conditions. The higher the elevated LDL cholesterol and triglyceride levels and the lower the HDL cholesterol levels, the greater the risk.

3: Blood Glucose

Blood sugar levels are another consideration. Elevated blood glucose promotes oxidative stress which subsequently damages blood vessels. Therefore, ensuring fasting blood glucose levels remain in the normal range of 70 to 100 mg/dL helps to reduce risk of cardiovascular and cerebrovascular diseases. The higher the fasting blood glucose and Hemoglobin A_{1C} levels, the greater the risk.

4: Physical Activity Level

Physical activity is beneficial on a variety of levels. First, regular moderate- or vigorous-intensity physical activity helps to burn calories and increase metabolism, which reduces excess weight and prevents weight gain. Second, regular physical activity protects against LDL oxidation by increasing antioxidant enzymes. Third, regular physical activity over time helps to increase HDL cholesterol, which in turn serves to remove the bad LDL cholesterol. Finally, physical activity has been shown to reduce psychological stress and blood pressure.

5: Diet

Consumption of foods high in sugar, salt, and saturated fat contributes to one or more of the conditions mentioned as risk factors earlier and in previous chapters. For example, dietary patterns high in salt can increase blood pressure. Excessive sugar can drive up insulin levels and promote weight gain. In addition, dietary intake of foods high in saturated fat and dietary cholesterol are associated with increased LDL cholesterol. A diet rich in vegetables, fruits, whole grains, and legumes has been shown to prevent, stop the progression, and in some cases even reverse cardiovascular and cerebrovascular diseases.

6: Weight

Maintaining a healthy weight helps to reduce the risk of cardiovascular and cerebrovascular diseases. A body mass index greater than 25 kg/m² with a waist circumference of >95 cm (37.4 inches) for men, and >80 cm (31.5 inches) for women increases the risk.

7: Tobacco Use

Quitting smoking (and use of other tobacco products) is something most every smoker will say they want to do, though this is easier said than done. Numerous studies over the last several decades link smoking to several diseases, including cancer, and cardiovascular and cerebrovascular diseases. Smoking promotes inflammation through harming the cells that line the interior walls of blood vessels, and promotes development of atherosclerosis by enhancing LDL oxidation.

When thinking of lifestyle and workplace environmental changes that may seem radical to us at the moment, we can gain perspective by keeping in mind that the detrimental effects of tobacco – something almost everyone now agrees is harmful – was once a controversial issue in the 1960s and 1970s. This controversy was largely shaped by lobbying and special interest groups fighting for tobacco's survival, despite the vast amounts of scientific research pointing to its harms. Some readers may recall the 1991 Journal of the American Medical Association study that found over 90% of 6-year-old children surveyed recognized the cartoon cigarette mascot Joe the Camel in relation to cigarettes.[92, 93] This was a wakeup call to parents and public health officials that tobacco companies might be marketing to children and starting them on an early path towards a dangerous, addictive habit. Since that time, tobacco's once behemoth influence has diminished to the point where companies not only institute smoking, and tobacco bans on company property, but also charge employees higher insurance premiums in many cases for using tobacco, and provide tobacco cessation support to employees interested in quitting. There are some companies that will no longer hire tobacco users due to the known dangers to health.

As I wrap up this chapter, I would be remiss to not point out that the current food environment of insulin raising ultra-processed foods, together with gigantic portions of artery clogging animal products, may very well be "the tobacco" of our era.

5 | ESTABLISHED DIETARY PLANS

There are four established dietary patterns that dietitians and nutritionists, as well as functional or lifestyle physicians, tend to recommend, and that nutritional researchers tend to study: The Whole-Food, Plant-Based (Vegan) Diet, The Ornish Diet, The Mediterranean Diet, and The DASH Diet. There is overlap between these diets in that they are all rich in whole plant foods, including fresh vegetables, fruits, whole grains, and legumes. However, there are varying degrees of "plant-basedness" among these diets. The Whole-Food, Plant-Based Vegan diet is entirely plant-based; the Dean Ornish dietary pattern is low-fat, high in complex carbohydrates and almost entirely plant-based with a few small animal-based exceptions; and the Mediterranean and DASH diets are more plant-based than the typical Western style diet but also comprise moderate portions of various animal products in the lean forms. All four of these dietary patterns have been associated with reducing chronic disease risk, and those that are more plant-based produce the best outcomes for reducing and even reversing chronic diseases.

The fifth dietary pattern covered in this chapter is what many people in more affluent countries follow, referred to here as the

"Western" style diet. This diet is high in saturated fat, dietary cholesterol, sugar, and salt, but is low in vegetables, fruits, whole grains, and fiber. This dietary pattern has been shown to be associated with promoting disease risk, and has been an important contributor to rising healthcare costs, reduced productivity, and adverse environmental impact on water, land, and greenhouse gases.

Whole-Food, Plant-Based Diet

A whole-food, plant-based vegan diet is devoid of all animal products, including eggs, dairy, and all terrestrial and aquatic animal flesh. Instead, it relies solely on vegetables, fruits, whole grains, legumes (beans, peas, lentils), nuts, and seeds. Every vitamin and nutrient the human body needs for growth, development, and cell function comes from the earth. More specifically, these fundamental nutrients are derived from the sun, the plants, and the soil in which plants grow. Most readers are undoubtedly familiar with the concept of a vegan diet, but it's important to clarify that a plant-based or vegan diet is not always "whole-food" (meaning minimally processed or unrefined) and thus not always a healthful dietary pattern. For example, a person could eat a diet of French fries, cola, coconut ice cream, and packaged cream sandwich cookies and still qualify as vegan, but most would agree that these foods alone do not constitute a nutritious dietary pattern. Therefore, including "whole-food" in the plant-based diet nomenclature allows for an important distinction. In what follows, I use the term "plant-based" to mean both "whole-food" and "plant-based."

Numerous epidemiological studies have looked at populations that eat a mostly or entirely vegetarian or vegan diet, and have compared them with those populations that do not. One of the more well-known is the Adventist Health Study and the follow-up Adventist Health Study 2 (AHS-2). Most of the research derived from these studies support the strong association between a plant-based (vegan) diet and reduced incidence of obesity and other chronic diseases. For example, in the study population of the AHS-2, researchers looked at four years of data from 22,434 men and 38,469 women. Different degrees of vegetarian diets were reviewed and further analyzed: vegan (consuming no animal products); lacto-ovo vegetarians (consuming eggs and dairy); pesco-vegetarians (consuming fish); semi-vegetarians (occasionally consuming animal products); and non-vegetarians (consuming typical quantities of animal products).[94] Vegans were the only group with a normal BMI and had a 62% reduction in the prevalence of type 2 diabetes compared to non-vegetarians[94]. As shown in Table 5.0, the study results suggest a positive association between BMI and prevalence of type 2 diabetes, corresponding also to an increase in consumption of animal products.[94] This means as more animal products are consumed, both BMI and type 2 diabetes rates tend to increase. This is referred to as a "dose-response" relationship.

Table 5.0: Adventist Health Study-2 results of 60,903 subjects, 2002 - 2006[94]

Measure	Vegan	Lacto-ovo Vegetarian	Pesco-Vegetarian	Semi-Vegetarian	Non-Vegetarian
BMI (kg/m^2)	23.6	25.7	26.3	27.3	28.8
Type 2 diabetes	2.9%	3.2%	4.8%	6.1%	7.6%

African Americans have historically suffered from disproportionally higher prevalence of type 2 diabetes than their European American peers. Four years after publishing their findings, the researchers in the aforementioned AHS-2 study looked specifically at the association between African Americans and various dietary patterns to see if there were different trends for this subset of the population.[95] They found a 78% reduction in the risk of type 2 diabetes among African American vegans compared to African American non-vegetarians, and after controlling for age and BMI, African American vegans still had a 62% reduction in the risk of type 2 diabetes compared to African American non-vegetarians.[95]

In a randomized clinical trial, over a 16-week period 75 participants who had excessive weight or obesity were divided into either the intervention group, where they followed a low-fat whole-food, plant-based diet, or the control group, where no dietary changes were made.[96] Low-fat meant less than 20% of daily caloric intake was fat. Additionally, the intervention group was not instructed to count calories or worry about how much food they ate; they could eat as much as they wanted. The aim of this study, published in 2018, was to look at pancreatic cell function and insulin resistance in subjects who did not have a history of diabetes.[96] The reader will recall from Chapter Three that under normal conditions, pancreatic cells release insulin in response to consumption of food containing carbohydrates. The carbohydrates are then broken down into glucose, where it is taken up by cells and used for energy. Therefore, assessing pancreatic cell function and insulin resistance can help clinicians predict an individual's risk of acquiring type 2 diabetes. The results of this study found that several biomarkers for type 2 diabetes and other chronic diseases improved in response to the plant-based, low-fat intervention diet. Specifically, after 16 weeks the intervention group exhibited reduced BMI, reduced visceral fat volume, reduced LDL cholesterol, reduced fasting plasma glucose, and improved glucose induced insulin secretion in comparison to the control group.[96] BMI decreased by 1.9 kg/m^2 for the intervention group but decreased only 0.2 kg/m^2 for the control group; visceral fat decreased 199 cm^3

for the intervention group but increased 25 cm³ for the control group; and fasting plasma glucose decreased 20.2 mmol/L for the intervention group but increased 16.0 mmol/L for the control group.[96] This study provides compelling evidence that a whole-food, plant-based diet can reduce the risk of type 2 diabetes.

Additional studies have been conducted using a whole-food, plant-based diet as treatment for one or more chronic diseases. In the BROAD study, published in 2017, researchers looked at the effect of a whole-food, plant-based diet on BMI and various metabolic markers for heart disease for a population in New Zealand who suffered from excessive weight or obesity and who had been diagnosed with type 2 diabetes, heart disease, hypertension, or dyslipidemia.[97] The intervention group was instructed to follow a low-fat, plant-based diet that included whole grains, legumes, vegetables, and fruits, and to avoid refined oils (e.g., olive oil, canola oil, coconut oil) and animal products.[97] Participants in the intervention group did not count calories, but instead were instructed to eat until they were full.[97] Meanwhile, the participants in the control group received "standard medical care."[97] Based on the data from 65 participants (33 in the intervention group and 32 in the control group), the intervention group exhibited statistically significant reductions in weight, BMI, LDL cholesterol, waist circumference, and hemoglobin A_{1c}, a measure used to diagnose type 2 diabetes.[97] The control group saw a slight reduction in LDL cholesterol, but no change in weight, BMI and waist circumference, whereas hemoglobin A_{1c} worsened.[97] See Figure 5.0. The data presented represents the percent change from baseline at three and six months for BMI (kg/m²), LDL cholesterol (mmol/L), waist circumference (cm), and hemoglobin A_{1c} (mmol/mol).

Creatinine, a measure used to assess kidney function improved for the intervention group; whereas there was no statistically significant change in creatinine for the control group.[97] Neither group saw a statistically significant change in triglycerides or blood pressure.[97] Finally, the intervention group participants were able to reduce their medication usage from a pooled 94 to 74 prescriptions for the whole group at six months (and further reduced medication usage to 67 prescriptions at twelve months), while the control group increased their medication usage from a pooled 74 to 80 prescriptions.[97] Since prescription medications make up a large part of employer healthcare costs, implementing a plant-based workplace could reduce this expense.

In another study, researchers looked at the effects of a low-fat, plant-based vegan diet on various metabolic factors in patients taking prescription medication for type 2 diabetes.[98] Ninety-nine participants were randomly assigned to either the low-fat vegan intervention group or a control group that followed the 2006 American Diabetes Association (ADA) dietary recommendations.[98] The macronutrient calorie distribution of the low-fat vegan diet consisted of 10% of calories from fat, 15% from protein, and 75% from carbohydrates, and was made up of vegetables, fruits, whole grains, and legumes.[98] Portion sizes were not restricted, so patients could eat until satiated if they chose to do so.[98] The American Diabetes Association diet included a 500–1,000 calorie deficit and a macronutrient composition that included up to 7% saturated fat, 15-20% protein, and 60-70% carbohydrates and monounsaturated fats. This diet also allowed up to 200mg of dietary cholesterol each day (note that only animal products contain dietary cholesterol, and also tend to be high in saturated fat).[98] To isolate the effect diet has on specific metabolic risk measures, all participants were asked not to alter their exercise habits during the study period.[98] A summary of the statistically significant results over the first 22 weeks of this study for participants whose diabetes medications remained unchanged can be found in Table 5.1.

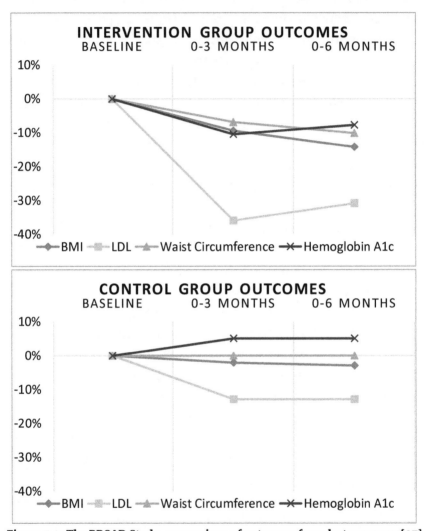

Figure 5.0: The BROAD Study, comparison of outcomes for select measures[97]

Table 5.1: Summary of results after 22 weeks of participants whose diabetes medications remained unchanged[98]

Measure	Low-Fat Vegan Intervention Group	ADA Control Group	Difference between Groups
Weight (kg)	-6.5	-3.1	-3.4
BMI (kg/m2)	-2.3	-1.1	-1.2
Waist (cm)	-5.0	-2.3	-2.7
LDL cholesterol (mg/dL)	-22.6	-10.7	-11.9
Total cholesterol (mg/dL)	-33.5	-19.0	-14.5

After 74 weeks, adherence to both diets waned, such that only 51% of the low-fat vegan diet group and 48% of the American Diabetes Association diet group continued to meet dietary adherence criteria.[99] Despite reduced adherence after 74 weeks, 35% of the low-fat vegan group and 20% of the American Diabetes Association group were able to reduce their diabetes medications in response to dietary changes.[99] While both groups exhibited improvements in various clinical measures, the low-fat vegan diet group saw greater benefits than the American Diabetes Association diet group, suggesting a dose-response relationship. More whole plant foods and fewer animal products were associated with better health outcomes in this study. There are numerous interesting conclusions to draw from this study, but most relevant to the issue of food environments in the workplace is this: why did the adherence to dietary instructions drop? Could it have been due to the study participants' obesogenic food environment? First, let us explore patterns beyond just the United States.

A 2016 Polish study looked at the cholesterol levels of 42 participants between the ages of 28 and 34 years old who were either omnivores or vegans.[100] There were no differences between the two groups in terms of BMI, waist to hip ratio, blood pressure, and heart rate.[100] What the researchers found was that LDL cholesterol and other concerning lipoproteins were lower in the vegan group. LDL was 79 mg/dL in the vegan group and 100 mg/dL in the omnivore group.[100] This effect may be due in part to phytosterols, which are found in plant-based foods and appear to have a cholesterol lowering effect in humans by reducing absorption of cholesterol in the digestive tract. [100] Now let's shift our attention to specific food groups.

It is common knowledge that whole grains are more nutritious than refined grains (white flour), but what does that have to do with disease risk and outcomes? There is a significant association between regular consumption of whole grains and reduced risk of colorectal cancer, for one.[101] Specifically, 90 grams of whole grains daily has been associated with a 17% reduced risk of colon cancer.[101] Ninety grams of whole grains is equivalent to 1¼ cup rolled oats (dry), ½ cup quinoa (dry), or ½ cup barley (dry). Furthermore, increased whole grain intake after diagnosis of colorectal cancer has been associated with an increased survival rate from this condition.[102]

What about the typical recommendation to eat more fruits and vegetables? A review of 95 different studies found that for every 200 grams of fruits and vegetables consumed daily, there is an 8-16% reduced risk in coronary heart disease, 13-18% reduced risk of stroke, and 3-4% reduced risk in total cancer.[103] Two hundred grams is roughly equal to 1½ cups of cooked vegetables, 3 cups of raw leafy greens, 1½ cups of blueberries, or 1½ large bananas.[104] Figure 5.1 shows the relative disease risk reduction associated with two levels of daily fruit and vegetable consumption.[103] As the reader will notice, the relative risk reduction associated with total cancer plateaus around 500g, but continues to increase for heart disease and stroke.

In an observational study conducted in Spain, researchers looked at fruit and vegetable consumption and blood pressure data from 4,393 participants.[105] The results showed an inverse relationship between prevalence of undiagnosed hypertension and the amount of vegetables and fruits consumed on a daily basis.[105].

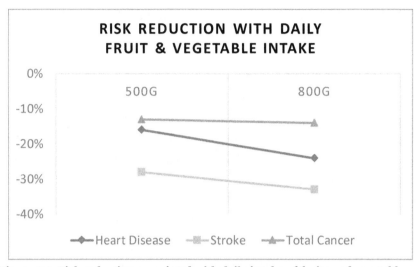

Figure 5.1: Risk reduction associated with daily intake of fruits and vegetables at 500g and 800g [103]

Legumes have been a food staple for people all over the world for thousands of years. Legumes include beans, lentils, and peas, and are high in protein, complex carbohydrates, fiber, and other micronutrients, yet are low in fat and contain no dietary cholesterol. For example, a cup of cooked black beans (240g) contains 218 calories, 15g protein, 1g fat, and 17g fiber, and is a good source of magnesium, potassium, phosphorus and folate.[104] Legumes are also inexpensive, have a long shelf life, and provide great versatility in meals with wide cultural culinary appeal (e.g., black beans in Latin America, chickpeas or garbanzo beans in Mediterranean countries, soybeans in Southeast Asia, and lentils in India). Legumes are also considered a resistant starch, which is the perfect substrate for microbes in the intestines to produce short chain fatty acids. As discussed in Chapter Two, these short chain fatty acids appear to play an important role in appetite regulation. In addition, regular consumption of legumes has been associated with lower LDL cholesterol and blood pressure, with positive implications for reduced risk of cardiovascular disease.

For those unfamiliar with what a whole-food, plant-based dietary pattern might look like, the rich variety of foods available can be surprising. Although many people on a whole-food, plant-based nutrition plan may eat elaborately prepared meals from time to time, such as Applewood Smoked Portobello or Lasagna Cruda from the award winning Plant Restaurant in North Carolina, the same pleasure is gained by eating simply, such as snacking on a piece of fruit or baby carrots, or, my personal favorite, eating an entire sweet red or yellow bell pepper. Furthermore, many of the most enjoyable whole-food, plant-based vegan meals are simple and affordable enough to be considered "peasant food," such as rice and beans seasoned with cumin and chili pepper, or cabbage, potatoes, and carrots seasoned with berbere spice. Table 5.2 outlines a sample meal plan of someone following a whole-food, plant-based vegan diet.

Many foods derived from animal products have plant-based substitutes. For example, cauliflower has been used as a pureed base for vegan alfredo sauce with whole wheat pasta, and is versatile enough to substitute for the "meat" in buffalo wings. Independent of the sauce, comparing cauliflower to the "meat" of chicken wings is enlightening. An entire head of cauliflower (medium size, 588g) is 147 calories, 12g fiber, 0.8g saturated fat, and 0mg cholesterol, whereas the same weight in chicken wings (588g) has 1,311 calories, 0g fiber, 26.2g saturated fat, and 447mg cholesterol. If calculated based on calorie percentages, both cauliflower and chicken wings have about the same amount of protein, comprising approximately 8% of total calories. For the same weight in foundational solid meal base we get nine times more calories, 33 times more saturated fat, no fiber, and a whole lot of cholesterol with chicken wings. There are several other plant foods commonly substituted for animal products, such as carrots used to make hot dogs; beets or portobello mushrooms used to make burgers; and tofu used to make ricotta cheese for lasagna or stuffed shells.

I would be remiss to end this section without a discussion of Vitamin B12. The only essential micronutrient absent from today's vegan diet is Vitamin B12, and therefore must be supplemented. Vitamin B12 is a water-soluble vitamin and is made in the gastrointestinal tract of animals by microorganisms found in residual soil or dirt in the food animals eat; picture a cow grazing on grass or a chicken scratching the ground to snatch up bugs. Vitamin B12 is then absorbed in the host animal, and in turn is assimilated by a human who eats the animal. If humans ate the dirt stuck to the carrots or potatoes coming out of the ground, they too would get Vitamin B12. However, since the soil is not as pristine as it may have once been several hundred years ago, and can also be hard on tooth enamel, most experts advise thoroughly washing vegetables and fruits before consuming, and instead supplementing the vegan diet with Vitamin B12.

Table 5.2: Whole-food, plant-based vegan meal plan examples

Meal Plan 1	Meal Plan 2
Breakfast	*Breakfast*
Steel cut Irish oats with chopped dates, fresh berries and ground flaxseed	Whole grain toast topped with almond butter and sliced banana
Snack	*Snack*
Green smoothie: coconut water, kale, cucumber, banana and ice, blended	Orange or grapefruit
Lunch	*Lunch*
Grilled veggie and roasted red pepper hummus wrap with whole wheat tortilla A side garden salad with garlic tahini dressing	Mixed greens salad topped with quinoa, carrots, cucumber, red onion, sunflower seeds, and balsamic vinaigrette Lentil chili, whole wheat pita
Snack	*Snack*
Sliced apple with peanut butter dip	Baked sweet potato with cinnamon
Dinner	*Dinner*
Black bean sweet potato and spinach enchiladas topped with cashew cream sauce and guacamole	Chana masala topped with chopped fresh cilantro and side of whole grain jasmine rice

Dean Ornish Diet

The Ornish Diet is a meal pattern low in fat and high in complex carbohydrates. It consists of whole foods – unprocessed or minimally processed and primarily plant-based – but also allows for small servings of egg whites and non-fat dairy (e.g., yogurt, skim milk). Besides the small exception of select animal products, another difference between the Ornish diet and the whole-food, plant-based vegan diet is that the latter includes fats from nuts, seeds, avocado and plant-oils, while the Ornish diet avoids or significantly limits these fats. Dr. Dean Ornish and his team of researchers conducted a study called The Lifestyle Heart Trial that was published in *The Lancet* in 1990.[106] This was groundbreaking work in that it was the first randomized controlled trial that looked at how lifestyle changes can reverse coronary heart disease without the use of cholesterol lowering medication.[106]

The experimental group ate a plant-based diet with a macronutrient composition of 10% calories from fat, 15–20% from protein, and 70–75% mainly complex carbohydrates.[106] In addition to the diet, the experimental group was also given meditation (stress reduction) protocols, exercise prescriptions (180 minutes moderate intensity per week), and group support, while the control group was simply asked to follow standard advice from their physician.[106, 107] After a 12-month period, there was a 37.4% reduction in LDL (bad) cholesterol in the experimental group compared to a 5.8% reduction in the control group, but no change in HDL (good) cholesterol for either group.[106] "Patients in the experimental group reported a 91% reduction in the frequency of angina (chest pain), a 42% reduction in duration of angina, and a 28% reduction in the severity of angina. In contrast, the control group patients reported a 165% rise in frequency, a 95% rise in duration, and a 39% rise in severity of angina."[106] After one year, 82% of the experimental group also experienced reversal of atherosclerosis compared to 42% of the control group.[106]

In 1998, Dr. Ornish and his team published a follow-up study to look at the sustainability of his program from the first study. After 5 years of following the lifestyle changes of eating a low-fat, high complex carbohydrate vegetarian diet, the experimental group experienced a 20% reduction in LDL cholesterol from baseline, while most in the control group began taking cholesterol medications and experienced twice as many cardiac events while following traditional advice from their physicians over the five years.[107]

Dr. Dean Ornish's diet and lifestyle intervention program, aptly called the "Ornish Reversal Program," has established credibility among insurers both private and public. Private insurers such as Anthem, Blue Shield of California, and Aetna, in addition to Medicare, are now willing to cover patients with coronary heart disease, and in some cases are covering those with other conditions, such as type 2 diabetes and prostate cancer, if they take measures to adhere to the Ornish diet.[108]

When some people think about a low-fat, high complex carbohydrate vegetarian diet, they may think of unpalatable foods that are more like tree bark and grass, but nothing could be further from the truth (although wheatgrass shots *are* popular among those looking for a nutrient-dense boost). A sample meal plan obtained from the Ornish website includes a variety of whole plant foods with small servings of egg whites and non-fat dairy. Cooking methods do not recommend use of oil, instead encouraging small amounts of nonstick cooking spray. Another technique that can be used is called dry sautéing, whereby a few tablespoons of water or vegetable broth is used instead of oil. Also, high fat plant foods such as nuts, seeds, and avocado are used sparingly, if at all. For example, there is a recipe for "Edamole" which uses high protein, low-fat edamame in place of avocado, which is traditionally used to make guacamole. See Table 5.3 for sample meal plans from the Ornish website. How does the reader's own workplace food environment stack up to these food items?

Table 5.3: Sample meal plans from Ornish.com website

Meal Plan 1	Meal Plan 2
Breakfast	*Breakfast*
Egg white vegetable frittata	Tofu scramble
Garlic roasted potatoes	Country sweet potatoes
Fresh strawberries	Sliced melon
Snack	*Snack*
Non-fat Greek yogurt, peaches, low-fat granola	Seasonal fruit parfait
Lunch	*Lunch*
Field greens salad with balsamic vinaigrette	Confetti citrus salad
Lentil chili	Smokey bean tacos with corn
Cornbread	Edamole
	Smokey chipotle sauce
Snack	*Snack*
Sliced cucumber, carrots	Sweet pea herb dip
Hummus (low fat)	Low fat whole grain crackers
Dinner	*Dinner*
Leafy greens salad with Italian dressing	Field greens salad with lemon miso dressing
Spinach & mushroom lasagna	Thai vegetable curry
Roasted asparagus	Brown jasmine rice
Cocoa truffles	Minted pineapple

Mediterranean Diet

The Mediterranean diet, like the DASH diet discussed in the next sub-section, includes variations that distinguish it from the diets discussed thus far. While this dietary pattern is omnivorous, it is still rich in whole plant foods. Also, "Mediterranean diet" is a loose category that contains several variations of its own. There are some Mediterranean dietary patterns with a more plant-based slant, such as what has been defined as a "traditional Mediterranean diet," in contrast to others that have less of a plant-slant, such as that defined by the United States Department of Agriculture, which the Department calls the "Healthy Mediterranean-Style Pattern," an adaptation from the "Healthy U.S.-Style Pattern."

Researchers in a 2003 observational study published in the *New England Journal of Medicine* described the traditional Mediterranean diet as "high intake" of vegetables, legumes, fruits, nuts, unrefined cereal grains, fish, and olive oil; a regular but moderate intake of wine with meals; a low-to-moderate intake of dairy products, typically cheese and yogurt; and a low intake of meat and poultry.[109] Researchers looked at adherence to this dietary pattern among a large sample of the Greek population using a 9-point scale (with higher numbers meaning greater adherence) from an extensive food frequency questionnaire and its relationship to mortality from certain disease conditions.[109] The researchers used the median intake of specific food groups to quantify high versus low adherence to the traditional Mediterranean diet, with high being more plant-based and low being less plant-based. Using data over a 44-month period of 22,043 participants, the results showed that high adherence to the traditional Mediterranean diet was associated with 25% reduction in mortality.[109] More specifically, for participants who were most faithfully adherent to a plant-based diet plus fish, there was a 37%

and 24% reduction in death from coronary heart disease and cancer, respectively.[109]

The United States Department of Agriculture (USDA) has outlined what it calls the "Healthy Mediterranean-Style Pattern," which is derived from its general "Healthy U.S.-Style Pattern." However, this pattern has less of a plant-slant than the traditional Mediterranean diet described above. For example, comparing similar daily caloric intakes, the USDA pattern suggests 2½ cups of vegetables each day, while stronger adherence to a traditional Mediterranean diet involves eating more than 3¼ cups each day. Using dairy intake as a gauge, the USDA pattern suggests 2 cups of dairy per day, but stronger adherence to a traditional Mediterranean diet indicates less than 1¼ cups of dairy per day. Given the USDA's objective to promote the economic interests of U.S. agriculture, including animal agriculture, it makes sense that any recommended dietary pattern promoted by the agency will necessarily include some components of dairy, meat, and eggs. The agency seems to be walking a fine line between promoting health and promoting the commercial interests of animal agriculture. After all, the USDA has been behind the most well-known TV commercial programs to promote some of the unhealthiest agricultural commodities: "Pork, the other white meat", "Beef, it's what's for dinner", "Got milk?," and "The incredible edible egg."

Table 5.4 summarizes plant-based foods common in the traditional Mediterranean dietary pattern that comprise the largest intake, whereas dairy, meat, and eggs are consumed in small amounts. Aquatic meat sources are also common in the traditional Mediterranean diet, and usually include: fish, shellfish, crustaceans and cephalopods.[110] How does the reader's workplace food environment stack up to these food items?

Table 5.4: Traditional Mediterranean foods eaten in abundance[110]

Food Category	Examples
Grains	barley, buckwheat, bulgur, farro, millet, oats, polenta, rice, wheatberries, breads, couscous, and pastas
Vegetables	artichokes, arugula, beets, broccoli, Brussels sprouts, cabbage, carrots, celery, celeriac, chicory, collard greens, cucumbers, dandelion greens, eggplant, fennel, kale, leeks, lemons, lettuce, mache, mushrooms, mustard greens, nettles, okra, onions (red, sweet, white), peas, peppers, potatoes, pumpkin, purslane, radishes, rutabaga, scallions, shallots, spinach, sweet potatoes, turnips, zucchini
Fruits	apples, apricots, avocados, cherries, clementine, dates, figs, grapefruits, grapes, melons, nectarines, olives, oranges, peaches, pears, pomegranates, strawberries, tangerines, tomatoes
Legumes, nuts & seeds	almonds, cannellini beans, chickpeas, cashews, fava beans, green beans, hazelnuts, kidney beans, lentils, pine nuts, pistachios, sesame seeds, split peas, tahini sauce, walnuts

DASH Diet

DASH is an acronym for "Dietary Approaches to Stop Hypertension" and was popularized after the results of a study published in the January 2001 issue of *The New England Journal of Medicine*.[111] The quality of this study was arguably higher than most in terms of validity and providing causal evidence. It was published at a time when the link between sodium intake and hypertension was coming to the forefront of general public awareness with mainstream media reporting the findings. I myself can remember going out and stocking up on Mrs. Dash's (unrelated to the DASH study) no sodium seasoning blend to sprinkle on my food around this time. The DASH diet is described as being "rich in vegetables, fruits, and low-fat dairy products," but also includes whole grains, poultry, fish, and nuts, as well as small amounts of red meat, sweets, and sugar-sweetened beverages.[111]

The DASH study took 412 participants who were not taking anti-hypertensive medication, and randomly assigned them to either eat the DASH intervention diet or the control diet.[111] The control diet was what the typical American adult consumed, which was (and still is) high in dietary cholesterol and saturated fat, largely from animal sources, and high in processed and refined grains and sugar.[111] Among each of the groups, participants were further randomly assigned to eat either a high, intermediate, or low sodium diet for a 30-day period.[111] The results of the study showed that even at the high sodium intake levels, the DASH diet participants significantly lowered their blood pressure more than the control diet; and similar results, but to a lesser degree, were seen at the intermediate and low sodium intake levels as well.[111] What this study revealed is that although excessive sodium intake can increase blood pressure, changing dietary composition to be more plant-based than animal-protein-based, irrespective of sodium levels, can still lower blood pressure.[111] Figure 5.2 graphically presents the difference in both systolic and diastolic blood pressure between the DASH diet and control diet at low, intermediate and high sodium intake levels.[111]

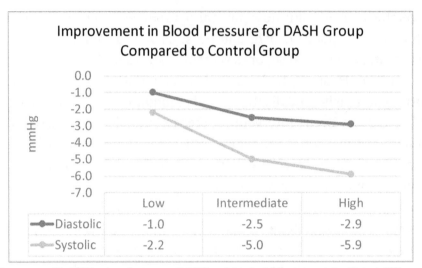

Improvement in Blood Pressure for DASH Group Compared to Control Group	Low	Intermediate	High
●Diastolic	-1.0	-2.5	-2.9
◉Systolic	-2.2	-5.0	-5.9

Figure 5.2: Net difference between DASH and typical Western style diet at different sodium intake levels[111]

The DASH diet is like the Mediterranean diet in that there are varying degrees of plant-slant in this general dietary pattern category. In general, the DASH diet prescribes consuming five cups of combined fruits and vegetables each day; three servings of whole grains per day; favors eating fish, poultry, and low-fat dairy in lieu of red and processed meats; limits sugar-sweetened beverages to no more than 36 ounces per week; and limits sodium to no more than 1.5g per day. In Table 5.5, there are two sample meal plans taken from the DASHDiet.org website, with the first one representing a non-vegetarian version and the second one representing the vegetarian equivalent. How does the reader's workplace food environment stack up to these food items?

Table 5.5: Sample DASH diet meal plans, non-vegetarian and vegetarian

Non-Vegetarian	Vegetarian
Breakfast	**Breakfast**
Oatmeal with applesauce Whole wheat English muffin with jam Low-fat yogurt Pineapple juice	Whole wheat cereal Nonfat milk Raspberries Orange juice
Lunch	**Lunch**
Chicken Waldorf salad Dinner roll Baby carrots Nonfat milk Cantaloupe	Santa Fe lentils in whole wheat or corn tortillas Side salad with ranch dressing Nonfat milk Pineapple slices
Snack	**Snack**
Light string cheese and kiwi	Reduced fat cheese and plum
Dinner	**Dinner**
Roasted chicken breast Baked potato Asparagus Tomato spinach salad with balsamic vinaigrette Apple crisp with frozen yogurt	Faux pasta e fagioli alla Venezia Stone fruit salad Glass of red wine

Anecdotally, I followed the non-vegetarian version of the DASH diet for years, sometimes taking in more than the recommended 2.3g of sodium in a day. While I did not have hypertension during that time, I still had borderline high cholesterol, suggesting that this dietary pattern, while better than the Western-style diet described next, still may not be good enough to check all the chronic disease prevention boxes.

The "Western" Style Diet

The "Western" style diet, sometimes referred to as the Standard American Diet, is characterized as high in saturated fat, cholesterol, refined grains, and sugar – basically, everything shown to increase disease risk. Concomitantly, it is low in vegetables, fruits, legumes, and whole grains. According to the USDA, cheese makes up the majority of saturated fat consumed in the United States, and its consumption has increased threefold since 1970. Altogether, the average American consumes 23 pounds of cheese each year. Table 5.6 summarizes the top 10 sources of American dietary saturated fat comprising half of all saturated fat consumed, based on data from National Health and Nutrition Examination Survey (NHANES)[112]:

Table 5.6: Top 10 sources of saturated fat in the U.S. diet (NHANES)[112]

Ranking	Food Item	Contribution to Intake (%)	Cumulative Contribution (%)
1	Regular cheese	8.5	8.5
2	Pizza	5.9	14.4
3	Grain-based desserts	5.8	20.2
4	Dairy desserts	5.6	25.8
5	Chicken, chicken mixed dishes	5.5	31.2
6	Sausage, franks, bacon, ribs	4.9	36.2
7	Burgers	4.4	40.5
8	Mexican mixed dishes	4.1	44.6
9	Beef, beef mixed dishes	4.1	48.7
10	Reduced fat milk	3.9	52.6

The average American added sugar intake is 23 teaspoons per day for children and adolescents; and 21 teaspoons per day for adults. For the average American adult, more than half of all added sugar intake comes from sodas and energy or sports drinks (at 37.1%), and grain-based desserts (at 13.7%). For children and adolescents, 31.8% comes from sodas and energy or sports drinks, while fruit drinks make up 15% of added sugar sources.[113] The vending machines and cafeterias often supply a plethora of added sugar in the form of sugar sweetened beverages, pastries, and other sweets. The foods employees consume at work may very well extend to a comparable dietary pattern in the home where children have access and form their habits.

Trans fats occur naturally in some foods (such as meats and dairy), but can also be industrially produced in a laboratory process known as hydrogenation for purposes of extending the shelf life of the product. Hydrogenation has been used by food manufacturers to make products containing unsaturated fatty acids solid at room temperature (i.e., more saturated) and, therefore, more resistant to spoilage and rancidity. Partial hydrogenation means that some, but not all, unsaturated fatty acids are converted to saturated fatty acids. Because numerous studies have shown that consumption of trans fats from partially hydrogenated oils are linked to cardiovascular disease, food manufacturers and restaurants have been pressured to reduce the amounts of artificial trans fats in many foods in recent years.

In 2015, the U.S. Food and Drug Administration announced it would no longer allow trans fats from partially hydrogenated oils after June 2018 without being granted special approval from the agency. However, to meet this requirement, many food manufacturers have replaced partial hydrogenation with full hydrogenation and then blending such oils with vegetable oils through a process called interesterification. Because this is a recent change, scientists do not fully understand the metabolic implications of interesterification on cardiovascular health. The only way to know if a product contains hydrogenated oils is to carefully read the ingredients label on the back of the package. Furthermore, many of these high fat processed foods also tend to be addictive and promote binge eating in certain people with obesity.[114] Given the addictive nature of these products and the fact that they still harbor ample amounts of saturated fats, added sugar and salt, it's probably best to rid the workplace of these types of snacks.

In 2015, the World Health Organization caused quite a stir. Based on a comprehensive review of the data, the International Agency for Research on Cancer (IARC), the cancer research agency of the World Health Organization, added processed meats to the list of class one carcinogens, ranking it as carcinogenic alongside the likes of asbestos and tobacco.[115] Yes, processed meats, including hot dogs, bacon, and sausage were now considered carcinogenic. When this was first published some healthcare providers were upset that the World Health Organization demonized processed meats, perhaps because they didn't want to give up their bacon. However, based on the body of evidence, the World Health Organization found that eating the equivalent of two breakfast sausage links a day would increase risk of colorectal cancer by 18%; and that the more a person eats, the greater the risk.[115] They went on to say that minimally processed red meat "probably" causes cancer too but stopped short of putting it on that dreaded list.

As mentioned, the Western style diet is low in vegetables and fruits. The recommendations from the 2015-2020 Dietary Guidelines for Americans is to consume between 1½ and 2 cups of fruit and 2 to 3 cups of vegetables each day. A 2015 Centers for Disease Control and Prevention Morbidity and Mortality Weekly Report, reports that of the over 373,000 American adults surveyed, 87% did not meet vegetable intake recommendations, while 76% did not meet recommendations for fruit intake.[116] The survey included a breakdown for each state, showing that only 5.5% of adults in Mississippi are meeting vegetable intake recommendations that and only 7.5% of adults in Tennessee are meeting fruit intake recommendations.[116]   The authors noted, "Substantial new efforts are needed to build consumer demand for fruits and vegetables through competitive pricing, placement and promotion in child care, schools, grocery stores, communities, and worksites."[116] I may be biased, but this sounds to me like a call to action for a plant-based workplace.

To summarize, the health promoting benefits of a plant-based diet are widely accepted among medical researchers and other scientists.   In fact, the Academy of Nutrition and Dietetics Association states in a 2016 position paper[117]:

> "...that appropriately planned vegetarian, including vegan, diets are healthful, nutritionally adequate and may provide health benefits for the prevention and treatment of certain diseases. These diets are appropriate for all stages of the life cycle, including pregnancy, lactation, infancy, childhood, adolescence, older adulthood and for athletes. Plant-based diets are more environmentally sustainable than diets rich in animal products because they use fewer natural resources and are associated with much less environmental damage." [117]

The only research debate is in how much animal foods a person can consume before it causes harm. We've all heard some story of that one guy who is the grandfather of a friend's nephew's cousin's friend who ate bacon, eggs, and biscuits every morning for breakfast with steak, potatoes, and butter for dinner and lived to be 95. However, just like the anecdotal person everyone seems to have heard about who smoked a pack a day for 70 years and never got lung cancer, these legendary people were either incredibly lucky or have a rare genetic gift that most people do not possess.

Dan Buettner's *The Blue Zones* provides a solid "gut check" for assessing the general truths for dietary patterns. He identifies five locations around the world with the highest percentage of centenarians in their populations. These included Sardinia (Italy), Okinawa (Japan), Loma Linda (California), Nicoya (Costa Rica), and Ikaria (Greece). One of the common dietary threads in these locations where people lived the longest and a high quality of life was their mostly plant-based food sources.

When we put all the data and studies aside and look more broadly at which societies have thrived, we find a compelling counternarrative to that one guy so-and-so knows who survived despite detrimental health habits. Successful business leaders don't develop business plans around these types of one-off exceptions. Instead, we develop plans based on broader likelihood and probability of occurrence. This is why implementing a plant-based workplace makes good business sense.

6 | THE PLANET

Businesses and municipalities all over the world have been inspired to erect blue or green bins for people to drop their glass, aluminum, plastic, and paper waste into for recycling. Of course, no single empty bottle of sparkling water will make a difference. However, it is widely accepted that several small changes do add up to make what is hopefully a meaningful impact. Over the last few decades, businesses have also worked to implement ecofriendly features in offices, factories and warehouses, such as low-flow toilets, daylight harvesting lighting, and use of hybrid or electric vehicles. All these improvements help the cause of saving resources and reducing pollution. The same logic can be taken a step further by implementing a plant-based workplace. As more people choose to eat plant-based, fewer resources are used in terms of water and land, and greenhouse gas emissions are reduced.

Many businesses that design, manufacture, and sell products utilize a Life Cycle Impact Assessment (LCIA or LCA) tool and process to quantify the total environmental impact of their product. It's a cradle-to-grave, or complete lifecycle, view that includes the supply inputs of materials processing, design, and development, and assesses them all the way to a finished product in production that is then used by the end-user, all the way through to when the product is decommissioned and discarded. LCAs are used for a vast number of products, from batteries in household electronics to jet engines on commercial aircraft, and everything in between. The same LCA methodology has been utilized by environmental scientists to quantify the impact of animal agriculture (including meat, fish, dairy, eggs) compared to plant-food (vegetables, fruits, cereal grains, legumes, seeds, nuts) agriculture on the environment. Numerous studies have been conducted and the bottom line is: animal foods use more resources and harm the environment more than plant foods, and locally grown plant-based food is best. In what way and by how much?

In a 2017 meta-analysis, researchers pooled data from 742 food production systems of over 90 foods published in 164 LCAs.[118] Approximately 86% of the data come from agricultural systems in North America, Europe, Australia, and New Zealand; with an additional 9% from Asia, including China and Japan; and the remaining 5% from South America and Africa.[118] The researchers looked specifically at five measures to quantify the environmental impact from cradle to farm-gate. The study stopped at farm-gate since there was too much variability to effectively measure a pooled environmental impact after the product leaves the farm (e.g., transportation of foods to various wholesalers, retailers, and end consumers).[118] The five environmental impact indicators for this cradle to farm-gate analysis included:

1: Greenhouse Gases

Greenhouse gas emissions, measured in CO_2 (carbon dioxide) equivalents, including carbon dioxide, methane, and nitrous oxide.

2: Land Use

Measures of the amount of land used in food production, including land used to grow feed for livestock as well as the land used by livestock directly for grazing, roaming, and sleeping.

3: Energy Use

Fossil fuel energy use, including all activities on and off the farm related to food production.

4: Acidification Potential

Acidification potential in the soil, a measure of nutrient loading, including sulfur dioxide, nitrogen oxides, nitrous oxide, and ammonia, among others.

5: Eutrophication Potential

Eutrophication potential, a measure of nutrient runoff into waters, including measures for phosphate, nitrogen oxides, ammonia, and ammonium found in fertilizers.

Using the five indicators above, Figure 6.0 provides a breakdown of the environmental impact on foods from animal sources compared to foods from plant sources based on serving size. The results of this systematic review showed that ruminant meats (cows, buffalo, goats, lambs, and sheep) had environmental impacts between 20 and 100 times those of plant foods, while other animal products (poultry, fish, eggs, and dairy) had between 2 and 25 times.[118]

At the time of writing this book, there are 7.6 billion people on Earth, and despite declining growth rates since the 1950s, the global population is expected to surpass 11 billion by 2090. Since we do not have an infinite amount of natural resources, biodiversity and clean air are threatened by a growing population and demand for foods from animal sources. The current model is not sustainable.

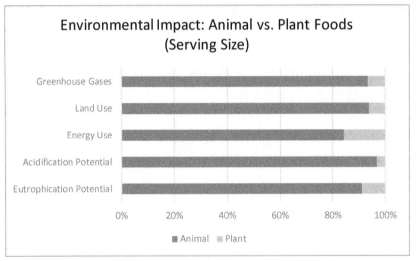

Figure 6.0: Breakdown of environmental impact, animal vs. plant foods based on serving size[118]

The next four sections in this chapter break down the major components of animal agriculture's impact on the environment, namely: greenhouse gas emissions, water depletion, land degradation, and threats to biodiversity. While I separately present each of these factors for further explanation, it is important to keep in mind that they are interconnected.

Greenhouse Gas Emissions

Greenhouse gases are the molecules in the atmosphere that trap and absorb radiation from the sun and contribute to climate change (also referred to as global warming). The gases of concern include carbon dioxide (CO_2), methane, and nitrous oxide. The U.S. National Oceanic and Atmospheric Association reported in 2013 that global carbon dioxide emissions reached record levels at 400 parts per million, and that "today's rate of increase is more than 100 times faster than the increase that occurred when the last ice age ended."[119] Animal agriculture is estimated to account for 14.5% of the total greenhouse gas emissions.[120]

While carbon dioxide makes up the largest percentage of greenhouse gases, methane is 25 times more efficient at absorbing solar radiation than is carbon dioxide, and nitrous oxide is 298 times more efficient. Experts use the term "CO_2 equivalent" to normalize the effect of the different gases, referred to as Global Warming Potential.[121] Therefore, 1 kg of methane is equal to 25 kg carbon dioxide, and 1 kg of nitrous oxide is equal to 298 kg carbon dioxide.

Research has revealed that animal agriculture contributes to greenhouse gases in four different ways: (1) artificial fertilizers and farm equipment; (2) enteric fermentation by ruminants; (3) manure management; and (4) deforestation and desertification for feed production and processing.

Fossil fuels include petroleum, coal, and natural gas, and are generally considered nonrenewable sources of energy. In animal agriculture, fossil fuels are used to power farm equipment and to produce chemicals that artificially enhance soil fertility, inhibit weeds from growing, and guards against pests and diseases in soil used to grow feed for cattle. When comparing the fossil fuel requirements, the relative effect of meat protein production is 6 to 20 times that of vegetable protein.[122] Fossil fuels from artificial fertilizers and farm equipment account for an estimated 6% of the agricultural greenhouse gas emissions.[120]

Ruminant animals include cows, buffalo, goats, lambs, and sheep. When these animals eat, the carbohydrates they consume are broken down into simple molecules by microorganisms in the rumen (the first large compartment of the stomach) for absorption into their blood stream for use as energy. This fermentation process results in the emission of methane gases, mainly through belching with a smaller amount emitted through flatulence. Recall that 1 kg of methane is equal to 25 kg carbon dioxide, and imagine how this could add up. This enteric fermentation by ruminant animals accounts for an estimated 39% of the animal agriculture greenhouse gas emissions.[120]

Manure management is the process and system by which animal waste (manure) is captured, stored, and recycled. Manure is a large contributor to greenhouse gases because it emits both highly efficient nitrous oxide and methane. Nitrous oxide is produced when manure, as well as urine, which is high in ammonium, mixes with the soil; whereas methane, affected by temperature among other conditions, is created during the microbial anaerobic decomposition of organic matter in livestock feces and bedding material (e.g., straw).[123] Manure management accounts for an estimated 10% of the animal agriculture greenhouse gas emissions.[120]

Deforestation of land used for livestock grazing, as well as to grow feed, accounts for the largest component of animal agriculture greenhouse gas emissions, at just over 45%, in the form of carbon dioxide production.[120] Because trees contain significant amounts of carbon in their tissues, burning or cutting trees through deforestation causes release of all that sequestered carbon dioxide. As more land is cleared and used to grow livestock feed, or for livestock grazing, less land is available and what remains rapidly becomes unproductive (sometimes through desertification). This results in soil erosion and threatens biodiversity, as is further explained below. Figure 6.1 summarizes the four different ways animal agriculture contributes greenhouse gas emissions.

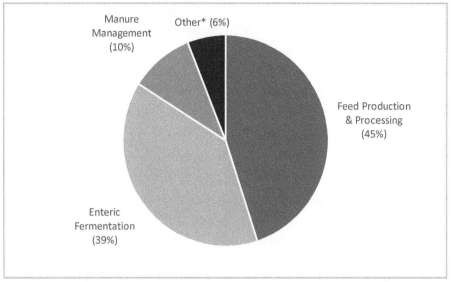

Other (6%) represents fossil fuels from artificial fertilizers and farm equipment

Figure 6.1: Four different ways animal agriculture contributes to greenhouse gas emissions[120]

Water Depletion

Water is essential to human life. In fact, it is the most important nutrient and required for our body's chemical processes. A human can live several weeks without food, but without water, the individual will likely die within a week. The importance of water and access to clean water is a major problem for a large percentage of the global population. I was listening to the Rich Roll podcast one afternoon while working out on my bike trainer. His guest was Scott Harrison, founder of a non-profit that brings clean, safe drinking water to people in developing countries.[124] He shared a story about a village in Ethiopia where young women are tasked with collecting water for use by the family. Starting their laborious journey at 4am, these women spend upwards of eight hours a day walking with a clay pot to collect water from the closest clean stream and then return to the village.[124] One day, a 13-year-old girl from a small Ethiopian village went to collect water for her family. They needed that water for the night's dinner, and before she returned home, she slipped on a rock, and dropped and broke the pot, losing that day's water.[124] She then committed suicide by hanging herself from a tree in shame because she lost the water and the $3 clay pot. Imagine this heartbreaking scene: she was just 13 years old.[124] Hearing this story caused me to stop pedaling, pause the podcast, and sit still on my bike while I processed what I had just learned. Like many people in developed countries, I took for granted the easy access to water that I've been afforded my entire life. How many times have I taken a longer-than-needed shower or unnecessarily left the water running while I was doing something in the kitchen? If 70% of total water withdrawals are for agriculture, while only 10% is used for industrial and 20% for personal use, why is there so much emphasis on efficient flushing toilets and shorter low flow showers? [125] Of course, we should all do our part to conserve water, but even more can be done through adoption of a plant-based diet.

About 98% of the water used for animal agriculture goes towards irrigation for grazing and crop production for livestock feed, while livestock drinking water and farm service water account for the remaining 2%.[126] That's right, we're using precious resources to water the grazing fields and gardens (corn, soybeans, and other grains) for animals to eat so that we can then eat the animals (flesh) or what they produce (eggs, dairy). The global water footprint of animal production is 2,422 cubic gigameters (Gm^3) per year and accounts for 29% of the total water footprint of 8,363 Gm^3 per year for total agricultural production in the world.[126] Converting cubic gigameters into cubic meters, 2,422 Gm^3 is 2,422,000,000,000 m^3 or 2,422,000,000,000,000 liters of water each year. The largest contributors are beef cattle (798 Gm^3

per year, or 33%); dairy cattle (469 Gm³ per year or 19%); pigs (458 Gm³ per year or 19%); and broiler chickens (255 Gm³ per year or 11%).[126] How do plant foods stack up against animal foods? In general, animal foods require more than twice as much water as plant foods to produce. Figure 6.2 illustrates the water footprint of various foods from both animal and plant sources.[126]

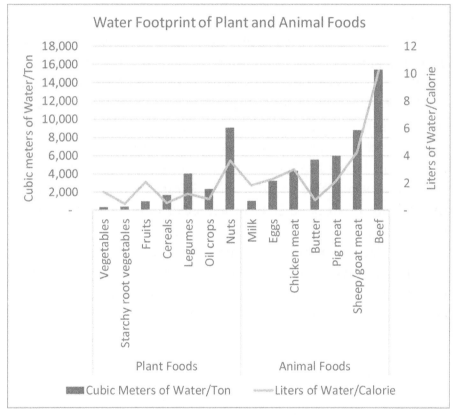

Figure 6.2: Water footprint of various plant and animal foods based on volume and energy contribution[126]

Solely from a water footprint standpoint, replacing pork, chicken or beef with heart-healthy, fiber rich legumes would save between 2 and 10 times more water for the same quantity of calories. Although food insecurity and water scarcity also involve geopolitical complexities, there is a lot of water being consumed and a lot of infrastructure built to irrigate land used for livestock that could go towards directly supplying humans, like the 13-year-old girl from Ethiopia and her family, with this basic nutrient essential to life.

Land Degradation

Land degradation is a broad term used to describe the decline in overall quality and use of land due to human activities or natural phenomena. There are several ways land degrades, including soil erosion, which is the removal or displacement of the top layer of soil adversely impacting land fertility; soil pollution, which involves the presence of contaminants from toxic chemicals and pesticides in the soil; desertification, where fertile land becomes desert and vegetation is not able to grow; and deforestation, which involves the clearing of trees such as in degraded rainforests, threatening biodiversity.

Most people's meat, milk, cheese, and eggs are sourced from concentrated animal feeding operations (CAFO), sometimes referred to as factory farms. Antibiotic use is necessary to reduce the spread of disease common when animals are confined in such close quarters. In addition to disease risks, antibiotics are also proven to promote growth in animals, which, in combination with other chemicals, explains why that chicken breast our moms used to buy when we were kids were a lot smaller than what we can now buy from any big box retailer. A 2015 study reports that 80% of all antibiotics purchased and used in the United States are for animal agriculture, and that farmers add it to animal feed.[127] The article was a "call to action" from and to the medical community for the government to intervene because healthcare providers were seeing the impact of this "inappropriate overuse of antibiotics" creating antibiotic-resistance among the humans eating said animals, resulting in longer hospital stays and even death from mutated bacterial infections.[127] After the medical community expressed widespread concern about the "excessive" use of antibiotics, the United States Department of Agriculture, through the U.S. Food and Drug Administration, established limits on levels of antibiotics used in animal agriculture.[128] What does all of this antibiotic use have to do with land degradation? The manure from animals treated with antibiotics contains antibiotic residue that then leaches into the soil and aquatic environments.[129, 130] Implementing a plant-based workplace both reduces the risk of antibiotic resistance from eating treated animals, as well as not contributing to land degradation associated with animal agriculture's use.

Threats to Biodiversity

Some readers may remember those 8mm films teachers showed in 6th grade science class that revealed how ecosystem components work together to give us life. They described how humans share this planet with different animals, plants, microorganisms, minerals, and elements, all of which are interconnected and beautifully synchronized in harmony like Tai Babilonia and Randy Gardner at the 1979 World Figure Skating Championships in Paris. With energy from the sun, plants use carbon dioxide and water to carry out photosynthesis in order to grow and become food and nutrients for others, including humans. In my head, I can almost hear the film narrator with his soothing deep voice explaining how all this works, along with the crackly music playing in the background as a flock of birds fly freely across the sky. I wonder what videos will be played in classrooms 20 or 30 years from now about our ecosystem, because we are abusing this planet to the point where it will likely become uninhabitable for future generations.

Threats to biodiversity exist both on land and in aquatic environments. Animal agriculture on land threatens biodiversity because of deforestation and desertification, as well as the release of various substances, such as emissions from phosphate rock, acidifying compounds, and copper pollution.

Land use for agriculture is decimating tropical rainforests and threatening the extinction of thousands of different species. Over the last several decades, "agricultural expansion is, by far, the leading land-use change associated with nearly all deforestation cases (96%)."[131] The consequences of this deforestation of the rainforest is chilling. Deforestation increases greenhouse gases, because fewer trees and plants means less absorption of carbon dioxide, less release of oxygen, and less rainfall and less water overall. Since much of the water used in animal agriculture depends on rainfall, having less would necessitate exploitation of other sources, such as finite ground and surface water stores, for grazing and livestock feed crops. Rainforests also provide about 20% of the oxygen we breathe, are home to 50% of all living things on Earth, and control the climate cycle for the entire planet. This precious land is being cleared at a stunningly high rate to make way for livestock feed crops and farms. Because published estimates are based on legally cleared lands, deforestation is purportedly higher because of illegal clearing. Based on satellite imagery published in *Geophysical Research Letters*, net forest loss totals 62%, mainly driven by tropical rainforest loss.[132] Using the data from this study, Figure 6.3 shows the change in forest area over two decades as measured by satellite imagery from the University of Maryland.[132]

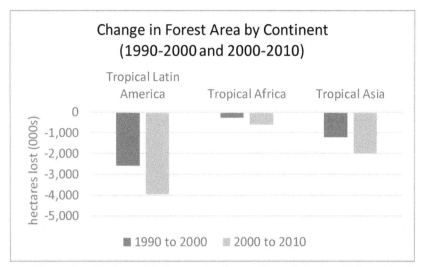

Figure 6.3: Net loss of deforestation by continent based on University of Maryland satellite images[132]

Why is there so much deforestation? Because people want to eat meat. With growing populations and rising incomes, demand for meat as food has increased. This is yet another reason to implement a plant–based workplace.

Synthetic fertilizer and livestock feed additives entail phosphate emissions that cause acidifying and eutrophic conditions, making land and aquatic environments uninhabitable for plants and certain animals. It has been estimated that meat production releases seven times more phosphate rock emissions than production of soybean vegetable protein.[122] Ammonia emissions, a byproduct of livestock waste, in addition to sulfur oxides and nitrogen oxides have created acidifying conditions and pH imbalances in surface waters and soil that dissolve the shells of aquatic organisms.[122, 133] Like phosphate emissions, these acidifying conditions are also causing eutrophication of surface waters, contributing to aquatic dead zones and declines in certain species.[133] Like the water, land is also susceptible to acidifying conditions. Meat production has been shown to emit seven times the amount of acidifying compounds as soybeans.[122] Part of this is due to trace minerals, such as copper, that are added to livestock feed and that are subsequently found in the manure of the animals. Adding copper and zinc to livestock feed helps prevent diseases, and possibly increases growth rates of livestock animals.[134, 135] These high concentrations of copper threaten soil and possibly biodiversity. A study conducted in China measured the concentration of copper in both feed and manure of different animals (i.e., pigs, cattle, chickens, and sheep). Results revealed that the highest concentrations came from pig and chicken manure at 699.6 mg/kg and 81.9 mg/kg, respectively.[134] It is widely accepted that copper toxicity injures plants and results in reduced growth, foliar chlorosis (iron deficiency), and abnormal or stunted root development.[136, 137]

A 2014 article in *Nature* entitled "Global diets link environmental sustainability and human health" provides lifecycle environmental impacts for different dietary patterns.[138] The article provides the greenhouse gas emission rates and net change in cropland reduction for the following diets: conventional omnivorous, Mediterranean, pescatarian (vegetarian plus fish), and a lacto-ovo vegetarian diet.[138] The per capita greenhouse gas reductions from the baseline omnivorous diet would be 30%, 45%, and 55% for Mediterranean, pescatarian, and vegetarian diets, respectively.[138] The net increase in land demand from 2009 to projected 2050 values (measured in 10^6 hectares), would be +590 for omnivorous diets, +130 for Mediterranean, +26 for pescatarian, and -16 for vegetarian.[138] Indeed, the authors forecast less future land use with a vegetarian diet. Although the authors did not quantify the impact of a whole-food, plant-based vegan diet, we can presume the greenhouse gas reductions would be greater than 55%, since eggs and dairy emit more greenhouse gases than vegetables, whole grains, and legumes; and land use reduction would be greater than -16 x 10^6 hectares, since the crop land needed to feed dairy cows could be excluded.

Threats to aquatic biodiversity involve over-exploitation of certain types of wild fish, as well as fish farming practices. Between 2007 and 2013, 30% of fish stocks were considered over-exploited.[139] Like terrestrial farming, farmed fish are penned in cages (not in the open waters), and subsist through the artificially provision of feed ingredients and antibiotics to combat diseases. However, some amount of medications and diseases are also transmitted through the waters to other aquatic life. The demand for fish continues to grow due to a surge in per capita consumption from 9.9kg in the 1960s to a record high of 20kg in 2014, coupled with the growing population.[139, 140] Aquatic biodiversity is also impacted by rising water temperatures, extreme weather events, and acidification from climate change. An increased prevalence of mass die-offs of fish and other aquatic animals has been reported in the news media, and experts attribute these mass mortality events to increases in diseases, biotoxicity, and other stressors, such as starvation, eutrophication-induced oxygen depletion, and extreme temperature changes.[141]

In summary, the interconnection of greenhouse gas emissions, water depletion, land degradation, and threats to biodiversity, both on land and in water, all centers on a growing human population, in which those with higher income levels want (but do not need) to eat more animal products. Again, 96% of deforestation activity – particularly of the precious tropical rainforest land where 20% of our oxygen is produced, and which serves as the regulator of global climate – is due to agriculture, threatening biodiversity and life as we know it on this planet. So, recycling that old stack of Harvard Business Review magazines piling up in the corner of the office or taking that shorter shower in the morning, while helpful, will not in and of itself save this planet; but I contend that if actions were also taken to reduce consumption of animal products by implementing a plant-based workplace, it will give us a fighting chance.

SECTION II: THE BUSINESS CASE

"In any moment of decision, the best thing you can do is the right thing, the next best thing is the wrong thing, and the worst thing you can do is nothing."

THEODORE ROOSEVELT,
26TH PRESIDENT OF THE U.S. (1858–1919)

7 | THE FINANCIALS

B efore we feel ready to start crunching numbers, we might wish to address the worry that if we implement a plant-based workplace, there is no guarantee employees will adopt a plant-based eating pattern outside of work, and all the hard work and effort to make this change could be undermined. But we can derive reassurance from the "dose-response" relationship discussed earlier. To illustrate this point, we can look to a 2013 study in which more than 200 employees at ten GEICO insurance sites participated in a randomized controlled trial over an 18-week period that measured how a plant-based nutrition program can reduce employee body weight and cardiovascular disease risk.[142] The total employee population was 20,000 and worksites were located in multiple geographical locations: Tucson, Arizona; San Diego, California; Lakeland, Florida; Macon, Georgia; Chevy Chase, Maryland; Buffalo, New York; Woodbury, New York; Dallas, Texas; Fredericksburg, Virginia; and Virginia Beach, Virginia.[142] After 80 people discontinued the study for various reasons (48 and 32 participants dropped out of the intervention and control groups, respectively), a total of 211 participants (or 1% of the total workforce) completed the full 18 weeks, with 94 in the intervention group and 117 in the control group.[142]

I found the lessons in this real-life plant-based workplace intervention encouraging. Specifically, even though dietary adherence to the low-fat, plant-based diet was mediocre at best, results still showed improvements in most biomarkers. The intervention group adherence to dietary cholesterol intake (≤50mg per day), total fat intake (≤25% of calorie per day), and saturated fat intake (≤5% of calories per day) were only 47%, 30%, and 29%, respectively.[142] Since low-fat vegan options were available and group support was provided at the workplace, lack of adherence may have happened when the employee was not at work. Or perhaps low adherence was due to the temptation posed by unhealthy foods coworkers ate in the presence of the intervention group, who may have "slipped" while at work. Despite the suboptimal adherence, the results were more favorable than not. Specifically, the intervention group saw reductions in weight, BMI, LDL cholesterol, and Hemoglobin A_{1c}; however, there were increases in triglyceride levels and decreases in HDL cholesterol.[142] Table 7.0 summarizes the changes in different variables of the 211 participants who completed the program.

Table 7.0: Summary of changes to clinical variables[142]

Clinical Variables	Intervention Group		Control Group	
	Baseline	18-Week (change)	Baseline	18-Week (change)
Weight (kg)	93.3	89.0 (-4.3)	93.5	93.4 (-0.1)
BMI (kg/m2)	33.5	32.0 (-1.5)	34	34.0 (0.0)
LDL cholesterol (mg/dL)	109	96 (-13.0)	110	108 (-2.0)
HDL cholesterol (mg/dL)	55	51 (-4.0)	56	56.7 (+0.7)
Triglycerides (mg/dL)	129	143 (+14)	127	124 (-3)
Hemoglobin A_{1c} %	7.52	6.78 (-0.74)	7.03	7.13 (+0.10)

These results provide additional evidence for the benefits of a plant-based workplace, but also suggest employees could benefit from nutrition education and support for making food choice decisions both within and outside the workplace. Ideally, widespread implementation of plant-based workplace food environments will set broader trends for community environmental changes that will then provide the positive feedback loops that enhance preference for plant-based foods in the workplace.

Now let's crunch some numbers. Profit losses associated with chronic disease conditions can be quantified based on direct medical costs and reduced productivity. Here I focus on the costs associated with obesity because is the initial condition that pave the way for the other comorbidities discussed in previous chapters. Direct medical costs comprise medical visits (office-based, hospital outpatient, hospital inpatient, emergency room, and home healthcare) and prescription medications, as well as medical supplies, devices, and related equipment. Productivity losses occur due to either absenteeism, in which an employee fails to show up to work; or presenteeism, in which an employee is present but is not able to work at full capacity due to illness or injury. Studies show that the business cost impact of presenteeism is significantly greater than that of absenteeism.[143, 144] In one study that looked at over 7,000 employed adults (18 to 65 years old), researchers define and measure presenteeism as "the average amount of time between arriving at work and starting work on days when a worker is not feeling well, and the average frequency of engaging in five specific work behaviors: losing concentration, repeating a job, working more slowly than usual, feeling fatigued at work, and doing nothing at work."[145] The specific question the researchers asked participants in order to quantify presenteeism was: "During the past seven days, how much did your health problems affect your productivity while you were working?"

Participants responded using a rating scale of 0 to 10, where 0 was "health problems had no effect on my work" and 10 indicated "health problems completely prevented me from working."[145] The results showed that 42% of workers with obesity reported health-related lost productivity time, compared to 36% of workers of healthy weight.[145]   Based on these results, researchers estimated the U.S. economic impact of lost productivity due to obesity to be $11.7 billion higher than it would have been had all workers been at a healthy weight.[145] To further explain how both direct healthcare costs and productivity are impacted, let's walk through a hypothetical example.

Alex, a 40-year-old male, works in the stockroom at a manufacturing plant in Michigan. His job is physical: he takes parts in from receiving and delivers them to the stockroom. When parts are needed, Alex physically moves them to the appropriate locations on the factory floor for use. He logs an estimated 3 to 4 miles of walking each day. Alex is 5 feet 10 inches tall and weighs 215 pounds (98 kg), placing his BMI at 30.8, which is considered obese. Alex was recently informed by his physician during a wellness visit that he also has hypertension. The doctor writes a prescription and tells Alex that he should eat healthier to lose weight, and that she wants to see him again in a month. The medical costs associated with Alex's obesity-related medical care will include all outpatient visits and the prescription for medication. The most commonly prescribed antihypertensive drug is Lisinopril.[146] Lisinopril is relatively inexpensive at a cost of $3.70 for a 30-day supply, and if Alex were the only employee to worry about, the fiscal impact might be negligible.   However, because of the high prevalence of hypertension, employers spend millions of dollars each year on even the most affordable antihypertensive drugs.   According to Statista.com, 116 million Lisinopril prescriptions were filled in the United States (in both private and publicly funded medical expenditures) in 2014, up from 58 million in 2004.[147] Medicare payments alone for Lisinopril totaled $319 million in 2015, covering over 85 million 30-day prescription fills.[148]

Let us return to Alex. In addition to his non-routine outpatient visit and medication, Alex's productivity would be adversely affected. The key risk factors of presenteeism for Alex would be the side effects of medications, as well as sleep disorders such as sleep apnea, which is common among people with obesity. The common side effects of the Lisinopril his doctor prescribed include blurred vision, tiredness, weakness, confusion, and lightheadedness.[146] Certainly, any one of these side effects, to say nothing of multiple side effects combined, will reduce Alex's productivity, as well as the productivity of those relying on him to move parts in the timely manner needed to meet customer delivery schedules.

I recall specific situations from when I was an operations manager for the plant in Mississippi in which employees had to take extra breaks or even had mood swings due to medication side effects. One employee even yelled at me for no apparent reason and later apologized, blaming his diabetes medication for his mood swings. Most of us can probably recall specific moments when someone in our work team had to leave work early or take a longer break, or when someone made more errors than usual, dozed off while at work, or experienced mood swings that disrupted employee relations. These real-life productivity killers add up to millions of dollars in company profit losses each year.

The cost impact of chronic disease on productivity is indisputable. A 2008 study involving 4,153 Shell Oil Company employees (median age of 47 years old) who were employed during the 10-year period spanning 1994 to 2003 at the Texas, Louisiana, or California refineries.[149] Of the 4,153 employees, 1,204 (or 29%) suffered from obesity (BMI $\geq$ 30 kg/m^2), and 1,854 (or 44.6%)

had excessive weight (BMI 25 to 29.9 kg/m²); and the researchers found that over the 10-year period, 31% to 36% of employee's lost work days were attributable to excessive weight and obesity.[149] Furthermore, the calculated annual direct costs due to lost work days was $405 and $933 per employee with excessive weight and obesity, respectively, totaling over $1.87 million in annual profit losses.[149]

Healthcare economists have published research on the cost of obesity and related comorbidities for several years now. The challenge in accurately estimating profit losses centers around deciding which data to use and which assumptions to make. Even systematic reviews or meta-analyses acknowledge the challenge of data heterogeneity.[150] However, at some point we must settle on one well-informed estimate to approximate profit impacts. I have selected one to use for illustrative purposes that I believe to be reasonable, if more conservative, than other possible estimates. Even if the estimate I have chosen underestimates the fiscal impact of chronic disease, it still proves sufficiently large to warrant the implementation of a plant-based workplace that promotes health and reduces the risk and prevalence of obesity and other chronic diseases.

The data summarized in Tables 7.1 and 7.2 are from a 2017 *Obesity Journal* study entitled "The Additional Costs and Health Effects of a Patient Having Overweight or Obesity: A Computational Model." The researchers utilized a Markov model – a randomly determined statistical process that measures the likelihood or probability of a series of events.[151] That is, even though obesity increases the risk of comorbidities, it does not guarantee that comorbidities will follow. In fact, a person with obesity can be metabolically healthy in terms of having normal blood pressure and normal blood lipids. In popular terms, this might be referred to as "healthy at any weight." However, on the other end of the spectrum, a person with obesity could also develop several comorbidities such as hypertension, diabetes, and dyslipidemia. The researchers used a model that takes into consideration both ends of this spectrum when deriving age-based cost estimates. [151] This model does not include all the additional comorbidities touched on in previous chapters of this book, such as osteoarthritis and cancer. In terms of costs, the analysis does not factor in absenteeism, nor the detriment to other coworkers imposed by the reduced productivity of the employee suffering from one or more chronic diseases. Thus, the cost estimates in this study could be construed as conservative, understating the true fiscal impact.

Table 7.1: Summary of cost estimates comparing excessive weight to normal weight ($US)[151]

Starting Age of Individual	Incremental Net Present Value of Lifetime Costs			Incremental Annual Average Costs		
	Medical	Productivity	Total	Medical	Productivity	Total
20	$5,055	5,358	$10,365	$114	125	$239
30	$5,130	6,019	$10,992	$155	197	$345
40	$5,452	7,651	$13,185	$252	388	$643
50	$5,866	10,205	$16,169	$444	847	$1,291
60	$5,702	12,582	$18,604	$668	1,518	$2,194
70	$5,177	12,098	$17,297	$960	2,239	$3,210

Table 7.2: Summary of cost estimates comparing obesity to normal weight ($US)[151]

Starting Age of Individual	Incremental Net Present Value of Lifetime Costs			Incremental Annual Average Costs		
	Medical	Productivity	Total	Medical	Productivity	Total
20	$14,059	14,141	$28,020	$311	322	$630
30	$13,713	13,999	$27,331	$393	423	$804
40	$15,024	16,400	$31,447	$589	698	$1,293
50	$15,925	20,120	$36,278	$906	1,267	$2,176
60	$13,342	21,472	$34,649	$1,106	1,924	$3,030
70	$10,472	18,949	$29,424	$1,304	2,487	$3,806

Nonetheless, these data provide the "first pass" theoretical impact of obesity on any company's profit and loss. To illustrate how the data could be used, let us explore a simple fictional scenario.

Scenario: Acme Manufacturing Corporation in the Deep South

Acme is a manufacturing company with 1,200 employees distributed across three plants in Louisiana (300 employees), Alabama (500 employees), and Mississippi (400 employees) where excessive weight and obesity rates are above the national average. Using data from the Behavioral Risk Factor Surveillance System (BRFSS) published on the CDC website, the excessive weight and obesity rates in Louisiana, Alabama, and Mississippi are presented in Table 7.3.[152] Based on the age ranges of its employees, Acme could estimate the theoretical profit impact of excessive weight and obesity to be approximately $1.18 million each year. Tables 7.3 and 7.4 present assumptions and calculations, quantifying the theoretical annual impact of overweight at $424,529 and obesity at $750,689.

Taking these chronic disease data into account could help Acme design a business strategy that includes providing employees with nutrition education led by a qualified consultant alongside the implementation of food environment changes. This would enhance employee access to the plant-based foods that prevent or reduce incidence of chronic disease, adding profits to the bottom line.

To summarize the financial business case, whether we use actual data from the company health surveillance system, as in the Shell Oil case study, or use epidemiological data similar to that of the 2017 *Obesity Journal* study, the successful implementation of a plant-based workplace food environment will yield both tangible and intangible benefits, including lower direct healthcare costs, increased productivity, and improved quality of life for employees.

Table 7.3: Theoretical cost of excessive weight for Acme Manufacturing Co.

			Louisiana Site		
Age Group	Number of Employees by Age Group	State Overweight Rate	Theoretical *FTEs Overweight	Incremental Cost per *FTE Overweight	Total Incremental Annual Cost of Overweight
20	10	33.7%	3.4	$ 239	$ 805
30	25	33.7%	8.4	$ 345	$ 2,907
40	85	33.7%	28.6	$ 643	$ 18,419
50	90	33.7%	30.3	$ 1,291	$ 39,156
60	80	33.7%	27.0	$ 2,194	$ 59,150
70	10	33.7%	3.4	$ 3,210	$ 10,818
	300		101.1		$ 131,255
			Alabama Site		
Age Group	Number of Employees by Age Group	State Overweight Rate	Theoretical *FTEs Overweight	Incremental Cost per *FTE Overweight	Total Incremental Annual Cost of Overweight
20	75	33.8%	25.4	$ 239	$ 6,059
30	100	33.8%	33.8	$ 345	$ 11,661
40	120	33.8%	40.6	$ 643	$ 26,080
50	125	33.8%	42.3	$ 1,291	$ 54,545
60	80	33.8%	27.0	$ 2,194	$ 59,326
70	0	33.8%	0.0	$ 3,210	$ -
	500		169.0		$ 157,670
			Mississippi Site		
Age Group	Number of Employees by Age Group	State Overweight Rate	Theoretical *FTEs Overweight	Incremental Cost per *FTE Overweight	Total Incremental Annual Cost of Overweight
20	55	34.0%	18.7	$ 239	$ 4,469
30	75	34.0%	25.5	$ 345	$ 8,798
40	95	34.0%	32.3	$ 643	$ 20,769
50	100	34.0%	34.0	$ 1,291	$ 43,894
60	70	34.0%	23.8	$ 2,194	$ 52,217
70	5	34.0%	1.7	$ 3,210	$ 5,457
	400		136.0		$ 135,604
			Acme's Theoretical Impact of Overweight		$ 424,529

*FTE: Full-Time Equivalents

Table 7.4: Theoretical cost of obesity for Acme Manufacturing Co.

			Louisiana Site		
Age Group	Number of Employees by Age Group	State Obesity Rate	Theoretical *FTEs Obesity	Incremental Cost per *FTE Obesity	Total Incremental Annual Cost of Obesity
20	10	35.5%	3.6	$ 630	$ 2,237
30	25	35.5%	8.9	$ 804	$ 7,136
40	85	35.5%	30.2	$ 1,293	$ 39,016
50	90	35.5%	32.0	$ 2,176	$ 69,523
60	80	35.5%	28.4	$ 3,030	$ 86,052
70	10	35.5%	3.6	$ 3,806	$ 13,511
	300		106.5		$ 217,475
			Alabama Site		
Age Group	Number of Employees by Age Group	State Obesity Rate	Theoretical *FTEs Obesity	Incremental Cost per *FTE Obesity	Total Incremental Annual Cost of Obesity
20	75	35.7%	26.8	$ 630	$ 16,868
30	100	35.7%	35.7	$ 804	$ 28,703
40	120	35.7%	42.8	$ 1,293	$ 55,392
50	125	35.7%	44.6	$ 2,176	$ 97,104
60	80	35.7%	28.6	$ 3,030	$ 86,537
70	0	35.7%	0.0	$ 3,806	$ -
	500		178.5		$ 284,604
			Mississippi Site		
Age Group	Number of Employees by Age Group	State Obesity Rate	Theoretical *FTEs Obesity	Incremental Cost per *FTE Obesity	Total Incremental Annual Cost of Obesity
20	55	37.3%	20.5	$ 630	$ 12,924
30	75	37.3%	28.0	$ 804	$ 22,492
40	95	37.3%	35.4	$ 1,293	$ 45,817
50	100	37.3%	37.3	$ 2,176	$ 81,165
60	70	37.3%	26.1	$ 3,030	$ 79,113
70	5	37.3%	1.9	$ 3,806	$ 7,098
	400		149.2		$ 248,610
				Acme's Theoretical Impact of Obesity:	$ 750,689

*FTE: Full-Time Equivalents

8 | THE ENVIRONMENT

Nowadays many businesses view their environmental and sustainability efforts from a reputational point of view; being perceived by customers and the broader public as socially and environmentally responsible is the right thing to do. This goes beyond mere legal and regulatory requirements, since having this socially responsible reputation is necessary to attract the best talent, especially from the Millennial generation workforce. I recall attending two different recruiting events at or near local universities, where almost every job-seeking student I spoke with asked the question, "What does your company do in terms of environmental sustainability?" This question was asked even before the questions "How much does the job pay?" and "Would I need to relocate?" Furthermore, companies that place a higher emphasis on environmental sustainability perform better financially than those which do not. A 2016 *Harvard Business Review* article provides an in-depth business case for sustainability and highlights: (1) The top 100 sustainable global companies realized significantly higher sales growth, return on assets, profit before taxes, and cashflow from operations; (2) Companies with "superior environmental performance" had a lower cost of debt by 40-45 basis points; and (3) Share prices were higher among top sustainability companies, even during the 2008 recession, resulting in an average of $650 million in incremental market capitalization per company.[153]

When I worked in operations, we regularly tracked various environmental and sustainability measures to assess the site's environmental impact. Measures such as energy consumption, greenhouse gas emissions, water use, recycling rate, and zero waste-to-landfill are common examples. However, I have yet to come across a company that includes the workplace food environment in its calculation of these measures. A group of environmental and sustainability researchers in Europe looked at the hypothetical impact of cutting meat, dairy, and egg consumption in half, replacing those products with plant-based foods.[154] The results of this analysis showed that the entire European Union would reduce nitrogen emissions by 40% (for a total greenhouse gas emission reduction of 25-40%), with 23% less land use per capita.[154] Even though this study only looked at the environmental impact of food from a regional point of view, the data are still relevant to our current discussion since the workplace is a microcosm of the broader community.

Running the numbers to assess environmental benefits of a plant-based workplace can be handled in a similar fashion to existing Environmental Health and Safety metrics any business tracks and manages through a scorecard. For example, companies can measure the environmental impact of high volume food items based on existing measures they may already be tracking, such as CO_2 equivalents. This will allow them to offset CO_2 levels by implementing a plant-based workplace. If a workplace cafeteria replaces a 151g (5.3oz) beef burger with an equivalent size veggie burger, the company can expect to offset approximately 1,800kg in CO_2 emissions, saving 3,500 liters of water per burger. If the goal is to move towards a completely whole-food, plant-based workplace, a company can simply measure the baseline starting point (baseline number of whole-food, plant-based options divided by the total food options) and track a percentage of plant-based food items towards the target goal level, knowing this transformation will contribute to a lighter carbon footprint. The company may also consider offsetting carbon emissions by sourcing vegetables and fruits from local and regional farmers, since these sources represent a lower carbon footprint due to shorter transport distances. For example, the company might set a goal of having 80% foods from local sources (say, less than 150 miles from the workplace). Other ideas for measuring environmental improvements are further discussed in Chapter 10.

In summary, whether businesses care about environmental sustainability because of concern for future generations, the reputation of the company, or to increase shareholder value, implementing a plant-based workplace can provide businesses an opportunity to raise the bar above typical environmentally conscious practices. Furthermore, when prospective candidates ask, "What does your company do in terms of environmental sustainability?" the response the business can proudly give is: "We've implemented a plant-based workplace."

9 | OTHER LEGAL AND ETHICAL CONSIDERATIONS

After President Barack Obama signed the 2010 Affordable Care Act (ACA) into law, there was subsequent growth in corporate wellness programs, and companies have struggled to implement incentive strategies that reward healthy behaviors and penalize unhealthy behaviors. Specifically, incentives have resulted in some unintended discrimination concerns. Through these programs, companies have been on shaky ground in relation to the Americans with Disabilities Act and Title VII of the Civil Rights Act of 1964 (Title VII), sometimes even violating these laws. One key issue is the term "voluntary" as it relates to participation in wellness programs.[155]

Specifically, corporate wellness programs, while legal under the ACA, have been shown to disparately impact people of lower income levels, certain racial minorities, and people with disabilities or chronic illnesses.[155] Under the Americans with Disabilities Act, discrimination occurs when an employer treats an employee less favorably on the basis of being mentally or physically differently abled. The punitive terms of some wellness programs, such as imposing surcharges (e.g., imposing additional costs for not meeting certain criteria), tend to violate Title VII, which "bans discrimination against an individual with respect to their compensation, terms, conditions or privileges of employment because of such individual's race, color, religion, sex, national origin..." by disproportionately harming racial minorities.[155] For example, because African Americans have a higher prevalence of hypertension, if a company were to impose a surcharge for not maintaining a healthy blood pressure level as part of a wellness program, it would impose a disproportionate financial burden on this racial group and therefore might violate one or both of these laws. In 2014, the Equal Employment Opportunity Commission (EEOC) filed a lawsuit against Honeywell International for its practice of providing incentive credits to employees who underwent biometric and anthropometric screenings, while implementing penalties and surcharges for those who did not.[155]

While the court ruled in favor of Honeywell, these types of lawsuits can be costly to companies and their reputations, making other companies skittish, because no company wants to be wrapped up in a legal battle that may implicate them in discriminatory practices. Instead, companies are more inclined to play it safe by not fully implementing incentives allowed for in the ACA. "This lack of clarity has left federal and state courts directionless, and facilitates inconsistent and unpredictable rulings that will mislead and confuse employers and employees."[155]

Incentives have a place in promoting healthy behaviors, and implementing a plant-based workplace would facilitate the very healthy habits businesses would like employees to adopt. And unlike the unintended effects of ACA era wellness programs, the issue of discrimination would be off the table so long as healthy food-pricing strategies do not disadvantage low-income employees. The Food Research and Action Center notes that healthy food options are unavailable or limited at best for individuals struggling to overcome socioeconomic barriers, putting these populations at "an inherent disadvantage in the battle for better health and well-being." Besides the ultra-processed food companies and others who profit from people being chronically sick, who specifically would be harmed by a plant-based workplace?

When I first proposed this concept of changing the workplace food environment to colleagues, they did not dispute the evidence that this change would both transform employee health and mitigate the company's environmental footprint, but did express skepticism over the impact this would have on employees' freedom of choice. Let's examine their concern for a moment.

In a typical workplace, there is a percentage of employees who consciously decide not to succumb to the tempting, mindless eating habits of the Western style diet. Instead, they bring their own healthy food into the workplace, because they recognize that there is no source in the workplace from which to choose health-promoting food. Yet no one seems to be concerned that the current workplace food model undermines freedom of choice for employees who wish to eat a healthy diet. Would it undermine freedom of choice to flip this narrative? If companies implement a plant-based transformation of the workplace food environment to improve employee health overall, those employees who still wish to eat unhealthy foods still have the right to pack their own lunches. As companies consider making this transition, they must ask whether the rights of the majority who have been conditioned to eat unhealthy foods are more important than the rights of the minority who are desperately hoping for a workplace venue from which healthy plant-based foods can be purchased. I suspect that even those employees eating the current offering of unhealthy foods would welcome a workplace shift toward foods that leave them feeling healthier and happier. This visionary take on freedom of choice complements the strong financial and environmental sustainability business case for transforming the workplace food environment.

In 2013, the *New York Times* published Michael Moss's article "The Extraordinary Science of Addictive Junk Food," in which Moss describes a meeting that took place in 1999 among CEOs and presidents of the leading food companies – Pillsbury, Nestle, Kraft (Nabisco), General Mills, Proctor & Gamble, Coca-Cola, and Mars – where these companies acknowledged receiving "heat" from public health experts and policymakers for the growing obesity trend, yet chose to change nothing about their practices.[45] Public discontent centered on the ultra-processed foods these companies produce, which are high in the sugar, salt, and fat that is so successfully marketed to the American palate. Moss states that after speaking with over 300 food scientists, marketers, and senior executives currently or formerly employed in the processed food industry: "What I found, over four years of research and reporting, was a conscious effort – taking place in labs and marketing meetings and grocery-store aisles – to get people hooked on foods that are convenient and inexpensive."[45] This push toward product optimization, which included adding sugar or high fructose corn syrup to pretty much every product in the effort to find the "bliss point" for consumers had nothing to do with enhancing food nutrition.[45] It was about employing the most talented PhDs, scientists, and marketers from the best universities to develop products and get people hooked for a predictable, recurring revenue stream. Another concept mentioned was the mastery of "sensory-specific satiety" that involves complex chemical formulas that are alluring to the taste buds without overwhelming the brain enough to signal the individual to stop eating.[45]

As the public learned from the Moss article, the practices these companies use are deceptive and coercive, preying on people who are pressed for time and need convenient food sources. I struggle to find the ethical difference between the methods applied by ultra-processed food companies and those used by predatory mortgage lenders that financially exploit consumers. These companies have used compensation structures to incentivize their most talented and highly educated employees to develop products that will generate massive sales (not healthful nutrition). Our companies' employees – who are working hard to carry out their jobs as accountants, engineers, technicians, and programmers – are pitted against powerful food chemists and marketers. Rather than protecting employees from this predatory business model, we expect them to take personal responsibility for navigating a deceptive food system to figure out what is most healthful for them and their families.

In Chapter Five on dietary patterns, I discussed how strategic food labeling practices nearly conceal hydrogenated oils of ultra-processed food products found in many workplace vending machines. The label for these products are not only on the back of the package, but is also printed in such small print that most consumers would be unlikely to read the ingredients label paying for the product. Is this fair to the consumer? Can food product choice really be a matter of personal responsibility with these industry standards? Executives of processed food companies might feel a sense of pride in this genius product development strategy, achieved by a team of so-called "experts on cravings." However, in this case, marketing prowess becomes something that exploits consumers by maximizing sales of junk food to busy, stressed-out people who then become sick and cost businesses and taxpayers billions of dollars.

When we engage in cultural debates on freedom of choice, we might explore definitions of the word "freedom." *Merriam Webster Dictionary* defines freedom as "the various qualities or states of being free, such as: the absence of necessity, coercion, or constraint in choice or action; and the quality or state of being exempt or released from something onerous." How does freedom of choice play into individual health choices? Let us remember that half of American adults have one or more chronic diseases, and the prevalence grows to more than three-quarters for those age 55 and older. Knowing the role food plays in proliferation of these conditions, and given long-term dependence on pharmaceutical medications to live a longer, sick life, we might ask ourselves: is this what freedom looks like?

Going back to the workplace safety parallel, requiring employees to wear steel toe shoes in a factory that assembles 15-pound hydraulic motors does not undermine an employee's freedom to go home, slip on a pair of flip-flops, and drop a 15-pound dumb bell on their foot if they so choose. Having a plant-based workplace does not infringe on an employee's freedom to choose a Western style diet at home. It simply means that businesses cease supporting food environments that promote disease – and businesses are even in a position to help with broader health education and support, so employees can be successful in making similar changes at home if they choose. If those employees with chronic disease were to resist a plant-based workplace, they would be living a fantasy to imagine themselves free while beholden to a menu of prescription medications brought on by the very foods they might want to remain in the workplace. I believe this type of cognitive dissonance is the core reason many businesses have not yet changed their workplace food environment. In the name of freedom, many businesses are giving employees nothing but the right to easily get sick.

In summary, beyond the fundamental financial and environmental business cases for a plant-based workplace, the ethical considerations are equivalent to the moral obligation many business leaders feel to provide a safe workplace. The "Health" in EHS (Environmental Health and Safety) needs to be broadened to include all aspects of health, and not just acute health. Implementing a plant-based workplace does not take away someone's right to eat whatever they want; it's merely another way for businesses to show they care about the well-being of their workforce, while lowering healthcare costs, improving productivity and contributing to a food system that is more sustainable for our beloved planet Earth.

SECTION III: THE APPLICATION

"Perception is strong, and sight is weak. In strategy it is important to see distant things as if they were close and to take a distanced view of close things."

MIYAMOTO MUSASHI,
JAPANESE SWORDSMAN (1584-1645)

10 | APPROACHES TO CHANGING THE FOOD ENVIRONMENT

Food is a sensitive topic. It can be an emotional issue for people for many reasons. One reason pertains to our fundamental survival needs. In fact, food joins air, water, shelter, and sleep to make up the "Physiological Needs" base of the entire Maslow's Hierarchy of Needs pyramid. Food is also a culturally important topic in terms of types of foods attached to celebrations, life events, and traditions. Embarking on changing the workplace food environment requires sensitivity to these emotional aspects of food, which will be tough for some people to modify. When clients come to me – even athletes with dyslipidemia or pre-diabetes – it sometimes scares them to talk about eating more vegetables, fruits, whole grains, and legumes. This is not to say every client feels afraid. Some clients have actually responded with, "Tell me what I need to do and I'll do it." Understanding that there will be a spectrum of employee receptivity to workplace food environment changes is important when deciding how, what, and when to communicate, as well as when determining the rate at which workplace food changes are introduced.

Before diving into the mechanics of a change model, the overarching theme of transitioning to a plant-based workplace is best approached by authentically caring about others. Engaging employees requires inspiring those from multiple generations by painting a vision and mission that is connected to a higher social purpose. The vision and purpose are best communicated by starting with "the why." Specifically, letting employees know why it is important to transition to a plant-based workplace. Emphasizing the health benefits and potential for enhanced quality of life will appeal to Baby Boomers, while the Millennials will care deeply about the global ecosystem. Generation X employees will be concerned about both. This is not to say Baby Boomers don't care about the planet – they too care more and more, because their children and grandchildren will feel the effects of the changing climate. Also, Millennials, who assign great importance to work-life integration, will increasingly care about their own health as more and more observe older family members afflicted by the terrible consequences of chronic disease. There are certainly areas of overlap in what might motivate employee populations from different generations. Giving employees multiple reasons to care will inherently engage them in a holistic manner, unleashing the power of employees from all generations and resulting in successful change.

The Change Model

Implementing a plant-based workplace is a site-specific project or program – an important consideration if a business has a large campus or multiple sites in different geographic locations. Below are five high-level steps used with a "people change" management process that will help guide implementation of a plant-based workplace:

Step 1: Identify core team and executive sponsor

Step 2: Develop the plan

Step 3: Design communication, education, and training

Step 4: Inspire through engagement

Step 5: Measure, track, and adjust

Let's dive deeper into each step.

1: Identify core team and executive sponsor

Using a combined bottom-up and top-down approach, with middle management fully engaged, will facilitate participation and keep it aligned. Having spent a good chunk of my career in "middle management," I recognize that this is where change can either happen or fall apart, because it's where the cascade from the top meets the groundswell from the frontline.

The top-down starts with visible leadership from senior and middle management who walk the talk of what the business wants the food environment to reflect, whether it is a whole-food, plant-based vegan and Ornish diets, or a more DASH and Mediterranean-style diets. The final chapter of this book provides some ideas on setting the tone of the workplace food environment. The executive sponsor will own implementation of the plant-based workplace from start to finish, and will serve as a conduit between other leaders, middle management, and the core project team. This person should be influential, have a large scope of responsibility in the organization, and come across as enthusiastic about making the change. A caring and authentic leader will inspire employees and enhance the company's credibility when he or she can convey how a plant-based workplace further aligns the company's values with its behaviors.

The bottom-up approach starts with pulling a core team together that will have the duty of defining and implementing the plant-based workplace. If the business already has a wellness program in place – with established wellness coordinators, environmental sustainability teams, or employee resource groups – leveraging this existing infrastructure is usually the best bet. These individuals already have a passion for healthy eating and environmental sustainability, and know how to reach the target audience. The middle manager's role is critical to ensure that the right people are selected and freed up to serve on the core team. The middle manager may also be a member of this important team.

Ideally, the core project team includes a representative from the food supply chain (or the owner of food vendor contracts), EHS (environmental, health, and safety), human resources, and a representative from the frontline in addition to the manager. If possible, it helps to include a person from finance so metrics, budgetary and savings aspects can be addressed up front. It is important that each person knows why they are on the team, the role they fill, and how they can best contribute their unique area of expertise. To facilitate their collaborative work, one person needs to be designated core team leader. The company may also wish to bring in a consultant who has expertise in plant-based nutrition, as well as designing and implementing large-scale projects or programs to help this group. The strength and diversity of the group members will make for a strong team and successful implementation process. Depending on the size of the organization and whether members wear multiple hats, group size should be capped at 6 to 12 members.

This team will decide what the plant-based workplace will look like. Deliverables from this committee would likely include sample meal plans for the cafeteria, as well as proposed vending machine products. This committee should also provide guidance on how food pricing might work to help facilitate employee receptivity to the changes, together with complementary nutrition educational programs or campaigns. The group may also wish to come up with strategies that enhance engagement, such as organizing a "taste testing" event or two. In addition, the person from the organization responsible for food vending, such as the supply chain representative, will want to consider updating contract language to ensure compliance with the new plant-based work environment standards. If companies are under contract with vending and food service providers, the team should review and understand the current terms and conditions to determine how the change can be implemented. In these situations, the food vending company representative should not only be engaged, but also be an active member of the team. Depending on the restrictions in the contract, constraints may impact the timeline for implementation, but the team is encouraged to seek out some initial first steps within what is possible. If there is no contract or if the contract is nearing expiry, this team would help define the requirements for any RFPs (request for proposals) going out for bid, based on the future-state plant-based workplace. These requirements would need to include a variety of unprocessed or minimally-processed fresh and frozen whole foods that are plant-based. Special attention needs to be given to ensure appropriate nutrient-content with no excessive saturated fat, added sugar and salt.

The core team will also need to define the "people change" management plan. If the company already uses a specific change management plan model, it is best to go with that. Otherwise, a Prosci "Awareness, Desire, Knowledge, Ability, and Reinforcement" (ADKAR) model is best. All of the ADKAR components are needed to effectively manage the people side of change. A summary of each element follows.

- Awareness: Employees and managers are aware of the business reasons for change. Awareness is the goal and outcome of early communications related to an organizational change.

- Desire: Employees and managers are engaged and participate in the change. Desire is the goal and outcome of sponsorship and resistance management.
- Knowledge: Employees and managers know how to change. Knowledge is the goal and outcome of education, training and coaching.
- Ability: Employees and managers can realize or implement the change at the required performance level. Ability is the goal and outcome of additional coaching, practice, and time.
- Reinforcement: Employees and managers reinforce the change to ensure change sticks. Reinforcement is the goal and outcome of adoption measurement, corrective action, and recognition of successful change.

2: Develop the plan

Developing the plan involves diving into both the actual food environment change and the plan for how to manage the people side of the change. It is helpful if the core team sets aside 1 to 2 days to go through this planning, ideally using a face-to-face project start-up workshop approach. The core team leader should make every effort to work with the executive sponsor to ensure a well-organized project start-up workshop is conducted. This is an investment that will save time later. Prework for this workshop would include: (1) a clearly defined current state of the company's workplace food environment with available data and metrics (e.g., health-related, cost-related, and environmental sustainability-related) to understand the baseline; (2) clearance from core team members and their managers about serving on this team; (3) an established implementation budget from the executive sponsor; (4) clarity of scope; (5) reviewed copies of existing food vending contracts, identifying terms, conditions, and expiry; and (6) a clear agenda with deliverables. Figure 10.0 below is a sample agenda for illustrative purposes. It is not intended to be prescriptive, but rather to provide a sense of what the workshop might entail.

Plant-Based Workplace Project Start-Up Workshop Agenda

Day 1	Day 2
Executive Sponsor Kick Off	Refine Draft Future State PLant-Based Workplace w/Input from Executive Sponsor
Introductions & Ice Breaker	Brainstorm and define work breakdown structure
Review of Roles & Expectations	
Review & Analysis of Data (Health Surveillance System and Cost Estimates)	
Lunch	Lunch
Review & Analysis of Data (Environment-Sustainability)	Develop action plan with key owners and due dates
Review & Assessment of Food Vending contracts T&Cs	Develop first pass communication plan
Draft Future State Plant-Based Workplace	Agree to meeting cadence frequency and duration
Executive Sponsor Debrief – Day 1	Executive Sponsor Debrief – Day 2

Figure 10.0: Sample project workshop agenda

The key deliverables from the workshop would include a list of both acceptable and unacceptable foods for the future plant-based workplace; an estimated implementation budget; a concrete benchmark with clear measures; an action plan with each action item having one owner and a due date; a mechanism or process for handling questions or issues that arise; and an agreed-upon core project team meeting cadence, such as every Monday at 10:00am for one hour. This does not preclude the team from working together outside of scheduled meetings, but instead sets regular time aside to assess progress, work through issues and risks, as well as enable the executive sponsor to connect with the core team on a regular basis to keep his or her finger on the pulse and offer support. Alternatively, the core team leader may decide to have a separate meeting with the executive sponsor, depending on the company's standard procedure.

3: Design communication, education, and training

Messages to employees should occur according to the communication plan initiated at the project start-up workshop. This plan should address the following questions: Who is the audience? What is the messaging? Who delivers the message? How do they deliver the message? When do they deliver the message? What is the intended outcome of the communication? How will the company assess if the communication was successful or not? Because the project is fluid, the communication plan will also be designed in an iterative manner.

It may be important to plan for nutrition education and training, especially if the company does not already have a wellness program, or if an existing wellness program has not previously provided this type of training. If this type of training is needed, contracting with a qualified consultant, such as a nutritionist or dietitian trained in chronic disease prevention and plant-based nutrition, will help employees better understand why the company has chosen to implement a plant-based workplace. Providing this expert support may also inspire employees to incorporate similar dietary changes at home if they are currently following a Western style diet high in ultra-processed and fast foods, but low in vegetables, fruits, and other fiber-rich, nutrient-dense foods.

4: Inspire through engagement

Engaging employees to be an active part of the change can be highly effective in advancing progress. Companies can make it personal by having employees share why their health and quality of life is important to them and giving them the opportunity to post their stories in the office or on the factory floor. Perhaps a 55-year-old technician has young grandchildren she wants to see graduate college and get married one day. Sharing a picture of herself with her grandchildren on a workplace bulletin board would help her keep her focused on why she is taking control of her health through plant-based nutrition. Or maybe the 42-year-old mechanical engineer wants to retire early and travel the world. Posting photos of the places he wants to visit on the factory floor could help him keep his health goal in mind. Or perhaps there is a 28-year-old accountant who isn't thinking about health, but has photos showing the awesome beauty of the planet to remind him of the food sustainability goals he needs to meet for that beauty to endure. In addition to highlighting personal stories, conducting the aforementioned "taste tests" or focus groups to help finalize decisions between different plant-based food options can help draw people into the change and ensure that the company isn't wasting money on food employees won't be interested in purchasing.

Companies should have a realistic expectation about how long it might take employees to acquire a taste for whole plant foods. Relevant here is the term "mere exposure," coined in a 1968 research publication,[156] and suggests that repeated exposure to a given dietary stimulus will eventually enhance a person's receptivity towards it. In a small study of 24 male college students that exposed participants to a certain fruit juice, researchers found that the more frequently the juice was tasted, the more it was liked by the participant.[157]

Like these study participants, we can all think back to specific foods we disliked as a child or adolescent but now enjoy because we acquired a taste for them. Several years ago, I personally disliked the taste of mushrooms, but after repeated exposure to multiple types of mushrooms – cremini, white button, portobello, shitake – in diverse culinary applications, the unfamiliar fungi I once resisted have become one of my favorite foods to eat. This concept should be kept in mind when transforming the workplace food environment from one filled with highly palatable processed foods to one rich in more complex whole plant foods. Studies involving children indicate that it can take between 8 and 9 exposure events to begin to like a certain food.[158] I believe this to be true for adults as well, or perhaps even fewer exposure events. When I first tried kombucha probiotic tea, I found the cider vinegar flavor notes to be off-putting but kept trying different flavors because I knew the benefits to my gut and digestion were well worth it. By the fourth or fifth bottle, the crisp and tangy flavor of the cider vinegar became appealing to me.

5: Measure, track, and adjust

Just before the project launches, and then 30 to 45 days afterwards, it can be helpful to conduct a "lessons learned" capture. The core team should come together and go through the following 8 questions. There may be some overlap in the answers, and that's okay. Understanding the what and why – not just in the good, but also in the bad and just okay – will help the team make adjustments towards great.

1. What went well and why?
2. What could be done to make it go great?
3. What didn't go well and why?
4. What can be done to make it better?
5. What went just okay and why?
6. What do we continue doing?
7. What do we stop doing?
8. What do we change or do differently?

Transitioning to a plant-based workplace is like any other major workplace change a company has implemented. Whether a company has completed a kaizen process improvement event to reduce cycle time or has launched a new IT system to cut transaction costs, identifying the output signals of what the company set out to change is key to staying on track and knowing how well the change was executed. The benchmarks chosen should ultimately align to a broader business objective or goal. The measures identified during the project start-up workshop can be easily quantified and made visible on business and operational scorecards. In addition, ensuring people alignment, as well as accountability for seeing the transformation through, will include setting clear goals around individual and team performance plans. These goals and their targets are what serve as the basis for an employee or team's performance evaluation.

Many organizations use SMART goals to establish targets. SMART stands for specific, measurable, achievable, realistic, and time-bound. Below are three examples of goals and supporting actions.

1. Replace 3 regular items on the cafeteria menu to meet the DASH and Mediterranean style dietary patterns over the course of three months.
   a. Replace the sausage cheese breakfast sandwich with an egg white and spinach breakfast wrap on whole wheat tortilla.
   b. Replace sugar sweetened box cereal boxes with steel cut oatmeal and a side of dried and fresh fruit.
   c. Replace packaged cookies with seasonal fruit from local farmers.
2. Relocate the salad bar from the back corner to the front center of the cafeteria. Complete the project in six months and at or below budget.
   a. Replace two animal-protein options with two plant-protein options, such as a shelled edamame and quinoa, both of which are complete proteins.

    b. Implement a promotion to drive salad bar sales (e.g., a punch card that earns employees a free salad for every ten salads they buy).

3. Replace 50% of traditional vending machines offerings with fresh food options over the course of nine months.

    a. Start by removing the "worst offenders" – those items highest in added sugar; highest in sodium; and highest in saturated fat.

    b. Implement a "farmer's market" or Community Supported Agriculture program where employees can purchase fresh, locally grown produce.

    c. Partner with an existing vendor to find more suitable infrastructure options that offer fresh food vending.

If a company wants to make progress in getting people to eat more plant-based foods, but is not in a position to start replacing certain foods, considering how current foods are priced is a behavioral economics method companies can use to help kick-start the change in employee habits. This is an interim step to help employees prepare for the next change. If the company wants or needs to continue offering chili cheese hot dogs, and the workplace cafeteria can double the price of this menu item, and cut prices in half for the Mediterranean salad and veggie burger, then one would expect sales of hot dogs to decline, while salads and veggie burgers would increase. These tactics do drive behavior. Consider the soda taxes cities around the globe have imposed; these have been successful in getting people to drink more water and fewer sugar sweetened beverages. Employees may not be happy about it initially, but many will also understand the purpose of it (because the company will have already done a great job with nutrition education and preliminary communication), and in time will likely change their behavior to prefer the healthy option.

As discussed in Chapter Eight, it may be helpful to break down and post in food vending areas the environmental impacts for specific food items. Having a visual that shows employees how much water and land is saved, and how much greenhouse gas emissions are reduced, per food item purchased will help keep the spirit of the change visible for everyone. It may not be feasible to measure environmental impacts for every food item, so tracking the big hitters, and classifying them by "low," "medium," and "high" environmental impact might make more sense.

In summary, following the five-step process, along with using a "people change" management methodology such as ADKAR will increase the company's chances of successfully implementing a plant-based workplace.

If the reader is not the business leader or manager, but is an individual contributor who feels as passionate about changing the workplace food environment as I did back when I first approached the topic with the company for which I worked, I can offer three recommendations for changing the workplace food environment from the bottom up. First, set up a meeting with the manager to initiate dialogue, and encourage them and the person responsible for food vending to pick up a copy of this book. Schedule a follow-up meeting to have a constructive dialogue about what was learned, and brainstorm some options for the workplace. Be open to helping him or her test some small changes to see what sticks, and grow from there. Second, seek out like-minded individuals and start a regular plant-based potluck lunch at the workplace where the group discusses strategies for improving the workplace food environment. It could be weekly, monthly, or whatever works best for those who are interested. Publicize the group and be open to inviting anyone interested so those who may be "plant-curious" feel included to participate. Finally, make it personal and be the example that others are inspired to follow. Having a higher social purpose, and a deeper connectedness to something greater than ourselves, will attract others to want to get involved. Even if the group with these shared values and purpose is only a few people, remember Margaret Mead's famous quote: "Never doubt that a small group of thoughtful, committed citizens can change the world; indeed, it's the only thing that ever has."

11 | MAKING IT PERSONAL

In 2007, as part of a routine wellness checkup, I learned that I had high cholesterol and early signs of plaque building up in my arteries. The carotid artery scan report noted that I had the arteries of a 46-year-old, yet I was only 35. My doctor wanted to put me on the statin drug, Lipitor. I refused, telling him I was only in my 30s and I knew what I needed to do to take better care of myself. I told him I would eat healthier foods and work out more. His response was, "Well, that's not practical and I recommend you start this medication." I politely declined and walked out.

Even without the test results, I knew I wasn't consistent with physical activity and that my stress level was high, given the amount of traveling I did for my high-pressure job. Moreover, my husband and I were DINKs (dual income, no kids), and ate out a lot at nice steakhouses. Normal fare for us included the following: filet mignon with crème brûlée for dessert; chicken fajitas with flour tortillas, refried beans, and rice smothered with cheese; salmon filets with Hollandaise-topped broccoli and a baked potato loaded with butter and sour cream; or high-end burgers, sometimes with bacon, and a large chocolate milkshake to wash it all down. Unsurprisingly, around that same time my husband was diagnosed with atherosclerosis. He went to the hospital complaining of a "funny feeling in his chest" and after a few tests underwent balloon angioplasty and had two stents inserted into his arteries. He was only 47 years old. Afterwards, the cardiologist prescribed him a menu of pills, most of which he was expected to take for the rest of his life. To the cardiologist's credit, he did mention the Dean Ornish diet, but we just weren't ready to accept going completely plant-based, because we truly believed we couldn't give up meat, dairy, and eggs. Instead, we found a book from a Dr. K. Lance Gould that offered a middle-ground, which included some animal foods plus a "zig-zag" day. The dietary pattern outlined in Dr. Gould's book was something we could live with in light of my dyslipidemia and my husband's atherosclerosis. Looking back on that period, I now realize that our two health events were the beginnings of a wakeup call that took another five years to unfold.

From ages 36 to 40, I ate what I thought was a healthy diet that included chicken breast, cottage cheese, yogurt, skim milk, fish, eggs on weekends, and red meat about once per month. I also enjoyed vegetarian pizza loaded with cheese and veggie cheeseburgers. I was consuming between 3 to 4 servings of fruits and vegetables each day. During that period, I was following a version of the DASH and Mediterranean diets. My cholesterol numbers improved but were still borderline. More importantly to me, I just didn't feel well. I was tired, sluggish, and mentally foggy. I spent an entire year going on and off "detox cleanses" to gain more energy and hopefully drop a couple pounds in the process. I even tried a cleanse that included a concoction of lemon juice, cayenne pepper, and maple syrup for five days straight. (Hey, if Beyoncé did it, it must be a good idea, right?) I felt great after fasting when I used vegetable broth and fresh juice as the transition diet, but as soon as I returned to eating my normal "healthy" diet, I quickly felt sluggish again.

In January 2012, after the holidays and a decadent vacation in France, I decided to transition to a vegetarian diet. I set a goal of eating vegetarian twice a week for a month, then increased it to three times a week, and so forth until the transformation was complete. I was so gung-ho about it that I put it into my development plan at work and shared it with my team. This gradual approach gave me time to figure out my go-to meals and satisfying ways to substitute vegetarian ingredients for meat. It took me six months to fully transition, but in June 2012, I at last declared "I'm a vegetarian!" I was still eating a fair amount of low-fat dairy, as well as eggs. Only a few weeks into lacto-ovo vegetarianism, I came across two documentaries: *Forks Over Knives* and *Earthlings*. After watching both, I immediately went to my husband and proclaimed I was adopting a whole-food, plant-based vegan diet. Given his prior health events, he was completely on board with joining me on this new path. It was easy once I made the decision to do it since all I had to do at that point was remove dairy and eggs. It was by far the best decision I ever made for myself. I've had people ask me if I miss meat and dairy. Without hesitation, my response is an enthusiastic, "No!" I ate what most people eat for the first 40 years of my life, and I can say with confidence and conviction that nothing tastes as good as I feel today!

After only a few months of eating a whole-food, plant-based nutrition plan, my LDL cholesterol and triglycerides dropped over 23%, and I was no longer borderline. Now let's revisit the study I mentioned in Chapter One, in which a hospital employee study group showed no change in cholesterol after 15 weeks. What if the hospital had offered only whole-food, plant-based options? Would the 623 study participants have seen a reduction in LDL levels comparable to my own?

Given my own experiences and what medical research shows, it might seem counterintuitive for me to suggest that companies consider middle-ground DASH or Mediterranean diet food options for workplace food venues. While I am biased towards a whole-food, plant-based vegan diet, and the evidence supports this dietary pattern as superior in terms of leaving a lighter environmental footprint and sustaining a healthful life, there is good reason to also include the DASH and Mediterranean options. I view these two dietary patterns to be good gateway diets towards a later whole-food, plant-based nutrition plan. In my own case, it took five years from the start of my own health scare and my husband's stent procedure to fully transition to a whole-food, plant-based diet. Thus, I fully empathize with how difficult this change can be for many people. So much of our lives are centered around food. We derive comfort from reminiscing about Holiday dinners with family members who are no longer with us. Food is built into our culture and identity. However, the exciting thing I learned about adopting a whole-food, plant-based diet is that a person can discover new foods and flavors and create new traditions. After all, it's not really the food that binds us. It's the opportunity food provides us to bond with the people we love. Eating a whole-food, plant-based diet has given me the best chance of having more meaningful moments to collect over my lifetime.

The first step for a plant-based workplace can start with you. Regardless of your position in the company, being a visible leader and example is the best way to show others that you are walking the talk. If you are not an owner or manager, consider requesting a meeting with your supervisor to discuss your observations about the workplace food environment. If you currently eat a DASH or Mediterranean style diet, consider a 30-day whole-food, plant-based vegan challenge. Chronicle your journey using a blog or social media for others in your organization to follow. Share what you've learned and discovered, including the barriers and challenges and what you did to overcome them. If you're currently eating a

Western style diet, and not ready to go full-on whole-food, plant-based, then share what preliminary changes you are making towards a DASH or Mediterranean style diet. Perhaps you might switch out that Friday lunch cheeseburger and fries for a bowl of lentil soup and a mixed greens salad topped with a beautiful rainbow of vegetables. Even if you are still eating chicken or fish for dinner, you can model gradual change that can inspire healthy habits in your colleagues and employees.

In closing, our global food system is interconnected with the health of our bodies and of the planet. The food a company provides has profound implications for productivity, profits, employee well-being, and the global ecosystem. It is time to create a set of workplace food-environment standards analogous to other safety standards required for responsible business practices. In the end, it takes system thinkers to truly understand the gravity of what is at stake, and to do what will undeniably be accepted as the right thing to do.

ACKNOWLEDGMENTS

The pivotal point of my career change started with adopting a plant-based diet. Having my husband, Kevin Carter, jump on board so quickly can't be understated. So many big life changes, such as overhauling a diet, often fail because the spouse or family is not supportive of the change. I'm truly grateful for Kevin's enthusiasm to join me on the plant-based journey.

As I contemplated leaving my corporate job and transitioning into health and wellness, Dr. David Jones asked me a simple, yet thought provoking question: "Is your life a novel or an autobiography?" Meaning, was I writing my own story or was I letting someone else write it for me? Thank you, Dr. Jones, for asking me that question. At the same time, Mike Cobb was my cycling therapist – enduring hours of riding with me while I contemplated what to do. Thank you, Mike, for listening and offering your own story as perspective.

After I decided to write this book, I went through several iterations of book titles, scope of content to cover and overall flow. Thank you, Leslie Dunbar and Alison Carey, for offering your time to read my earlier versions of the manuscript, and give me feedback and critiques – it helped guide me towards this final product.

I can't begin to say enough about the amazing skills of my editor, Loretta Rafey. She exceeded my expectations in working to "fine tune and polish the marble" of my manuscript and delivered on all deadline commitments. Thank you, Loretta, you have been an absolute pleasure to work with and I'm grateful our paths crossed.

Thank you, Jay Iyengar and Paul Simon, for taking time out to read my manuscript, and for the thoughtfulness of your comments and feedback.

I was blown away when Dr. Joel Kahn took the time to read my manuscript and agreed to write the amazing foreword to this book. Thank you, Dr. Kahn.

Last, but not least, my mom. My mom who never stopped believing in me even when things weren't going well provided me with the emotional support to press forward. I love you, mom.

ABOUT THE AUTHOR

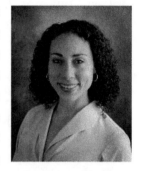

Gigi Carter was born and raised in Cleveland, Ohio and currently resides in the San Juan Islands in Washington state. She earned her bachelor's degree in economics from John Carroll University and a master's in business administration from Cleveland State University. Over the last 24 years, Gigi's career has been mostly with Fortune 500 companies in financial services and manufacturing leading and driving change. She's held management and leadership positions in finance and accounting, strategic planning, mergers and acquisitions, post-merger integration, operations management, project and program management, and operational and business process excellence. Gigi made a career change in 2016 to pursue her master's in nutrition sciences from the University of Alabama at Birmingham, where she graduated with honors, and launched a wellness coaching and consulting practice, My True Self, PLLC. Gigi is a licensed Nutritionist and certified personal trainer. Her focus area is with chronic disease prevention using plant-based nutrition and other lifestyle management concepts. When she is not working, Gigi enjoys spending time with her husband, Kevin, three rescued dogs and cycling.

REFERENCES

1. *Health*, in *Oxford English Dictionary*. 2018, Oxford University Press: Website.
2. *CDC's Chronic Disease Prevention System*. 2017 June 1, 2017 [cited 2018 January 1, 2017]; Available from: https://www.cdc.gov/chronicdisease/about/prevention.htm.
3. Saad, L. *The "40-Hour" Workweek Is Actually Longer -- by Seven Hours*. 2014 [cited 2017 December 16, 2017]; Available from: http://news.gallup.com/poll/175286/hour-workweek-actually-longer-seven-hours.aspx.
4. Bishop, K.B., E. Friedman, and M.G. Wootan, *Vending Contradictions: Snack and Beverage Options on Public Property*. 2014. p. 1-16.
5. Carrera, M., S.A. Hasan, and S. Prina, *The Effects of Health Risk Assessments on Cafeteria Purchases: Do New Information and Health Training Matter?* 2017: Case Western Reserve University. p. 1-58.
6. *Theory at a Glance* in *A Guide for Health Promotion Practice*, N.C. Institute, Editor. 2005, U.S. Department of Health and Human Services: National Institutes of Health. p. 52.
7. Stankevitz, K., et al., *Perceived Barriers to Healthy Eating and Physical Activity Among Participants in a Workplace Obesity Intervention*. J Occup Environ Med, 2017. **59**(8): p. 746-751.
8. *Climate Change and Biodiversity Loss*. March 15, 2018]; Available from: https://chge.hsph.harvard.edu/climate-change-and-biodiversity-loss.
9. *Livestock's Long Shadow: Environmental Issues and Options*. 2006: Rome.
10. *World population projected to reach 9.8 billion in 2050, and 11.2 billion in 2100*. 2017; Available from: https://www.un.org/development/desa/en/news/population/world-population-prospects-2017.html.
11. Kotter, J.a.C., Daniel, *The Heart of Change*. 2002: Harvard School Publishing.
12. Lake, A. and T. Townshend, *Obesogenic environments: exploring the built and food environments*. J R Soc Promot Health, 2006. **126**(6): p. 262-7.
13. Pincock, S., *Boyd Swinburn: combating obesity at the community level*. The Lancet. **378**(9793): p. 761.

14. Schulz, L.O. and L.S. Chaudhari, *High-Risk Populations: The Pimas of Arizona and Mexico.* Current obesity reports, 2015. **4**(1): p. 92-98.

15. Britannica, T.E.o.E., *Gadsden Purchase.* 2017, Encyclopædia Britannica, inc.

16. Ravussin, E., et al., *Effects of a Traditional Lifestyle on Obesity in Pima Indians.* Diabetes Care, 1994. **17**(9): p. 1067-1074.

17. Houmard, J.A., PhD, *Severe Obesity: Is there a metabolic program?*, in *NORC Seminar Series.* 2014, University of Alabama at Birmingham: Birmingham, AL.

18. *Assessing Your Weight.* 2015 [cited 2017 December 18, 2017]; Available from: https://www.cdc.gov/healthyweight/assessing/index.html.

19. *Waist Circumference and Waist-Hip Ratio: Report of a WHO Expert Consultation.* 2011: Geneva, Switzerland.

20. Ashwell, M., P. Gunn, and S. Gibson, *Waist-to-height ratio is a better screening tool than waist circumference and BMI for adult cardiometabolic risk factors: systematic review and meta-analysis.* Obesity Reviews, 2012. **13**(3): p. 275-286.

21. Lin, C.-H., et al., *Waist-to-height ratio is the best index of obesity in association with chronic kidney disease.* Nutrition, 2007. **23**(11): p. 788-793.

22. Caminha, T.C.S., et al., *Waist-to-height ratio is the best anthropometric predictor of hypertension: A population-based study with women from a state of northeast of Brazil.* Medicine, 2017. **96**(2): p. e5874.

23. Shen, S., et al., *Waist-to-height ratio is an effective indicator for comprehensive cardiovascular health.* Scientific Reports, 2017. **7**: p. 43046.

24. *Obesity: Situations and Trends.* Global Health Observatory (GHO) data [cited 2017 December 22, 2017]; Available from: http://www.who.int/gho/ncd/risk_factors/obesity_text/en/.

25. Dobbs, R., et al., *Overcoming Obesity: An initial economic analysis.* 2014, McKinsey Global Institute.

26. Hales, C.M., Carroll, Margaret D., Fryar, Cheryl D., Ogden, Cynthia L., *Prevalence of Obesity Among Adults and Youth: United States, 2015–2016,* in *NCHS Data Brief.* 2017, U.S. Department of Health & Human Services: CDC Website.

27. *The State of Childhood Obesity.* 2017 [cited 2018 January 4, 2018]; Available from: https://stateofobesity.org/childhood-obesity-trends/.

28. *Childhood Obesity Facts.* 2017 [cited 2018 January 4, 2018]; Available from: https://www.cdc.gov/obesity/data/childhood.html.

29. Fuemmeler, B.F., et al., *Parental obesity moderates the relationship between childhood appetitive traits and weight.* Obesity (Silver Spring, Md.), 2013. **21**(4): p. 815-823.

30.   Reilly, J.J., et al., *Early life risk factors for obesity in childhood: cohort study.* BMJ, 2005. **330**(7504): p. 1357.

31.   Trasande, L. and S. Chatterjee, *The Impact of Obesity on Health Service Utilization and Costs in Childhood.* Obesity, 2009. **17**(9): p. 1749-1754.

32.   Pulgaron, E.R. and A.M. Delamater, *Obesity and Type 2 Diabetes in Children: Epidemiology and Treatment.* Current diabetes reports, 2014. **14**(8): p. 508-508.

33.   Carey, F.R., et al., *Educational outcomes associated with childhood obesity in the United States: cross-sectional results from the 2011–2012 National Survey of Children's Health.* The International Journal of Behavioral Nutrition and Physical Activity, 2015. **12**(Suppl 1): p. S3-S3.

34.   Finucane, M.M., et al., *National, regional, and global trends in body mass index since 1980: Systematic analysis of health examination surveys and epidemiological studies with 960 country-years and 9.1 million participants.* Lancet (London, England), 2011. **377**(9765): p. 557-567.

35.   Ezkurdia, I., et al., *Multiple evidence strands suggest that there may be as few as 19 000 human protein-coding genes.* Human Molecular Genetics, 2014. **23**(22): p. 5866-5878.

36.   *GHRL gene.* Genetics Home Reference 2017 [cited 2017 December 29, 2017]; Available from: https://ghr.nlm.nih.gov/gene/GHRL.

37.   Müller, M.J., A. Bosy-Westphal, and S.B. Heymsfield, *Is there evidence for a set point that regulates human body weight?* F1000 Medicine Reports, 2010. **2**: p. 59.

38.   Martínez Steele, E., et al., *The share of ultra-processed foods and the overall nutritional quality of diets in the US: evidence from a nationally representative cross-sectional study.* Population Health Metrics, 2017. **15**: p. 6.

39.   Poti, J.M., B. Braga, and B. Qin, *Ultra-processed Food Intake and Obesity: What Really Matters for Health-Processing or Nutrient Content?* Curr Obes Rep, 2017. **6**(4): p. 420-431.

40.   *Ultra-processed foods are driving the obesity epidemic in Latin America, says new PAHO/WHO report.* 2015 [cited 2018 February 28, 2018]; Available from: http://www.paho.org/ocpc/index.php?option=com_content&view=article&id=408:2015-ultra-processed-food-drive-obesity&Itemid=1540.

41.   Canella, D.S., et al., *Ultra-Processed Food Products and Obesity in Brazilian Households (2008–2009).* PLOS ONE, 2014. **9**(3): p. e92752.

42.   Monteiro, C.A., et al., *Increasing consumption of ultra-processed foods and likely impact on human health: evidence from Brazil.* Public Health Nutrition, 2010. **14**(1): p. 5-13.

43.   Monteiro, C.A., et al., *Ultra-processed products are becoming dominant in the global food system.* Obesity Reviews, 2013. **14**: p. 21-28.

44.   Martinez Steele, E., et al., *Ultra-processed foods and added sugars in the US diet: evidence from a nationally representative cross-sectional study.* BMJ Open, 2016. **6**(3): p. e009892.

45.   Moss, M., *The Extraordinary Science of Addictive Junk Food*, in *The New York Times Magazine*. 2013, The New York Times.

46.   Asfaw, A., *Does consumption of processed foods explain disparities in the body weight of individuals? The case of Guatemala.* Health Econ, 2011. **20**(2): p. 184-95.

47.   Louzada, M.L., et al., *Consumption of ultra-processed foods and obesity in Brazilian adolescents and adults.* Prev Med, 2015. **81**: p. 9-15.

48.   Mendonca, R.D., et al., *Ultra-Processed Food Consumption and the Incidence of Hypertension in a Mediterranean Cohort: The Seguimiento Universidad de Navarra Project.* Am J Hypertens, 2017. **30**(4): p. 358-366.

49.   Williams, E.P., et al., *Overweight and Obesity: Prevalence, Consequences, and Causes of a Growing Public Health Problem.* Curr Obes Rep, 2015. **4**(3): p. 363-70.

50.   Barczynska, R., et al., *Dextrins from Maize Starch as Substances Activating the Growth of Bacteroidetes and Actinobacteria Simultaneously Inhibiting the Growth of Firmicutes, Responsible for the Occurrence of Obesity.* Plant Foods for Human Nutrition, 2016. **71**(2): p. 190-196.

51.   Chen, T., et al., *Fiber-utilizing capacity varies in Prevotella- versus Bacteroides-dominated gut microbiota.* Scientific Reports, 2017. **7**(1): p. 2594.

52.   Hjorth, M.F., et al., *Pre-treatment microbial Prevotella-to-Bacteroides ratio, determines body fat loss success during a 6-month randomized controlled diet intervention.* Int J Obes (Lond), 2017.

53.   Wansink, B.a.S., Jeffrey, *Mindless Eating: The 200 Daily Food Decisions We Overlook.* Environment and Behavior, 2007. **39**(1): p. 106-123.

54.   Chen, A. *Forcing People At Vending Machines To Wait Nudges Them To Buy Healthier Snacks.* Food for Thought 2017 March 31, 2017 [cited 2018 February 12, 2018]; Available from: https://www.npr.org/sections/thesalt/2017/03/31/522189753/forcing-people-at-vending-machines-to-wait-nudges-them-to-buy-healthier-snacks.

55.   Geier, A.B., P. Rozin, and G. Doros, *Unit bias. A new heuristic that helps explain the effect of portion size on food intake.* Psychol Sci, 2006. **17**(6): p. 521-5.

56. Vartanian, L.R., C.P. Herman, and B. Wansink, *Are we aware of the external factors that influence our food intake?* Health Psychol, 2008. **27**(5): p. 533-8.

57. Kuhnle, G.G.C., et al., *Association between sucrose intake and risk of overweight and obesity in a prospective sub-cohort of the European Prospective Investigation into Cancer in Norfolk (EPIC-Norfolk).* Public Health Nutrition, 2015. **18**(15): p. 2815-2824.

58. Jensen, M.D., et al., *2013 AHA/ACC/TOS Guideline for the Management of Overweight and Obesity in Adults.* Circulation, 2013.

59. *Physical Activity.* Global Strategy on Diet, Physical Activity and Health 2018 [cited 2018 January 3, 2018]; Available from: http://www.who.int/dietphysicalactivity/pa/en/.

60. Newman, E., D.B. O'Connor, and M. Conner, *Daily hassles and eating behaviour: the role of cortisol reactivity status.* Psychoneuroendocrinology, 2007. **32**(2): p. 125-32.

61. Torres, S.J. and C.A. Nowson, *Relationship between stress, eating behavior, and obesity.* Nutrition, 2007. **23**(11): p. 887-894.

62. Joseph, J.J. and S.H. Golden, *Cortisol dysregulation: the bidirectional link between stress, depression, and type 2 diabetes mellitus.* Annals of the New York Academy of Sciences, 2017. **1391**(1): p. 20-34.

63. Di Angelantonio, E., et al., *Body-mass index and all-cause mortality: individual-participant-data meta-analysis of 239 prospective studies in four continents.* The Lancet, 2016. **388**(10046): p. 776-786.

64. Spahlholz, J., et al., *Obesity and discrimination – a systematic review and meta-analysis of observational studies.* Obesity Reviews, 2016. **17**(1): p. 43-55.

65. Kitahara, C.M., et al., *Association between Class III Obesity (BMI of 40–59 kg/m2) and Mortality: A Pooled Analysis of 20 Prospective Studies.* PLOS Medicine, 2014. **11**(7): p. e1001673.

66. Basu, R. *Type 2 Diabetes.* 2017; Available from: https://www.niddk.nih.gov/health-information/diabetes/overview/what-is-diabetes/type-2-diabetes.

67. Kampmann, U., et al., *Gestational diabetes: A clinical update.* World Journal of Diabetes, 2015. **6**(8): p. 1065-1072.

68. Metzger, B.M. *Gestational Diabetes.* 2017 [cited 2018 January 3, 2018]; Available from: https://www.niddk.nih.gov/health-information/diabetes/overview/what-is-diabetes/gestational.

69. *Diabetes.* 2017 [cited 2018 January 4, 2018]; Available from: http://www.who.int/mediacentre/factsheets/fs312/en/.

70. *Statistics About Diabetes.* 2017 [cited 2018 January 4, 2018]; Available from: http://www.diabetes.org/diabetes-basics/statistics/.

71.   Bommer, C., et al., *The global economic burden of diabetes in adults aged 20–79 years: a cost-of-illness study.* The Lancet Diabetes & Endocrinology. **5**(6): p. 423-430.

72.   *The Staggering Costs of Diabetes.* 2017 [cited 2018 January 4, 2018]; Available from: http://www.diabetes.org/diabetes-basics/statistics/infographics/adv-staggering-cost-of-diabetes.html.

73.   Aubert, R., *Diabetes in America.* 2nd ed. Vol. Publication No. 95-1468. 1995: National Institute of Diabetes and Digestive and Kidney Diseases of the National Institutes of Health.

74.   *Diagnosed Diabetes* 2017 [cited 2018 January 4, 2018]; Atlas Data]. Available from: https://www.cdc.gov/diabetes/data/.

75.   *Your Weight and Diabetes.* 2015 [cited 2018 February 16, 2018]; Available from: http://www.obesity.org/content/weight-diabetes.

76.   Dabelea, D., et al., *Intrauterine exposure to diabetes conveys risks for type 2 diabetes and obesity: a study of discordant sibships.* Diabetes, 2000. **49**(12): p. 2208-2211.

77.   Jeon, C.Y., et al., *Physical Activity of Moderate Intensity and Risk of Type 2 Diabetes.* A systematic review, 2007. **30**(3): p. 744-752.

78.   Shinkman, R., *The Big Business of Dialysis Care*, in *NEJM Catalyst.* 2016, Massachusetts Medical Society.

79.   Whelton, P.K., et al., *2017 ACC/AHA/AAPA/ABC/ACPM/AGS/APhA/ASH/ASPC/NMA/PCNA Guideline for the Prevention, Detection, Evaluation, and Management of High Blood Pressure in Adults.* A Report of the American College of Cardiology/American Heart Association Task Force on Clinical Practice Guidelines, 2017.

80.   Muntner, P., et al., *Potential US Population Impact of the 2017 ACC/AHA High Blood Pressure Guideline.* Circulation, 2018. **137**(2): p. 109-118.

81.   *Understanding Blood Pressure Readings.* Know Your Numbers 2018 January 11, 2018 [cited 2018 February 11, 2018]; Available from: http://www.heart.org/HEARTORG/Conditions/HighBloodPressure/KnowYourNumbers/Understanding-Blood-Pressure-Readings_UCM_301764_Article.jsp.

82.   *Cholesterol Levels: What You Need to Know.* 2012 Summer 2012 [cited 2018 February 12, 2018]; Available from: https://medlineplus.gov/magazine/issues/summer12/articles/summer12pg6-7.html.

83.   *Triglyceride level.* 2018 [cited 2018 February 12, 2018]; Available from: https://medlineplus.gov/ency/article/003493.htm.

84.	*Hemorrhagic stroke.* 2018 March 15, 2018]; Available from: http://www.stroke.org/understand-stroke/what-stroke/hemorrhagic-stroke.

85.	*What You Should Know About Cerebral Aneurysms.* 2016 November 14, 2016 March 15, 2018]; Available from: http://www.strokeassociation.org/STROKEORG/AboutStroke/TypesofStroke/HemorrhagicBleeds/What-You-Should-Know-About-Cerebral-Aneurysms_UCM_310103_Article.jsp#.WqsHeujwY2x.

86.	*Heart Disease Facts.* Heart Disease Statistics and Maps 2017 November 28, 2017 [cited 2018 February 11, 2018]; Available from: https://www.cdc.gov/heartdisease/facts.htm.

87.	Salami, J.A., et al., *National trends in statin use and expenditures in the us adult population from 2002 to 2013: Insights from the medical expenditure panel survey.* JAMA Cardiology, 2017. **2**(1): p. 56-65.

88.	Mozaffarian, D., et al., *Heart Disease and Stroke Statistics—2015 Update.* A Report From the American Heart Association, 2015. **131**(4): p. e29-e322.

89.	*Raised blood pressure.* Global Health Observatory (GHO) data 2018 [cited 2018 February 5, 2018]; Available from: http://www.who.int/gho/ncd/risk_factors/blood_pressure_prevalence_text/en/.

90.	Gaziano, T.A., et al., *The global cost of nonoptimal blood pressure.* Journal of Hypertension, 2009. **27**(7): p. 1472-1477.

91.	Klein, R., et al., *Hypertension and retinopathy, arteriolar narrowing, and arteriovenous nicking in a population.* Archives of Ophthalmology, 1994. **112**(1): p. 92-98.

92.	Fischer, P.M., et al., *Brand logo recognition by children aged 3 to 6 years. Mickey Mouse and Old Joe the Camel.* Jama, 1991. **266**(22): p. 3145-8.

93.	Keck, K. *Big Tobacco: A history of its decline.* 2009.

94.	Tonstad, S., et al., *Type of Vegetarian Diet, Body Weight, and Prevalence of Type 2 Diabetes.* Diabetes Care, 2009. **32**(5): p. 791-796.

95.	Tonstad, S., et al., *Vegetarian diets and incidence of diabetes in the Adventist Health Study-2.* Nutrition, metabolism, and cardiovascular diseases : NMCD, 2013. **23**(4): p. 292-299.

96.	Kahleova, H., et al., *A Plant-Based Dietary Intervention Improves Beta-Cell Function and Insulin Resistance in Overweight Adults: A 16-Week Randomized Clinical Trial.* Nutrients, 2018. **10**(2): p. 189.

97.	Wright, N., et al., *The BROAD study: A randomised controlled trial using a whole food plant-based diet in the community for obesity, ischaemic heart disease or diabetes.* Nutrition &Amp; Diabetes, 2017. **7**: p. e256.

98.   Barnard, N.D., et al., *A low-fat vegan diet improves glycemic control and cardiovascular risk factors in a randomized clinical trial in individuals with type 2 diabetes.* Diabetes Care, 2006. **29**(8): p. 1777-83.

99.   Barnard, N.D., et al., *A low-fat vegan diet and a conventional diabetes diet in the treatment of type 2 diabetes: a randomized, controlled, 74-wk clinical trial.* Am J Clin Nutr, 2009. **89**(5): p. 1588s-1596s.

100.   Agnieszka Kuchta, A.L., Marcin Fijałkowski, Rafał Gałąska, Ewelina Kreft, Magdalena Totoń, Kuba Czaja, Anna Kozłowska, Agnieszka Ćwiklińska, Barbara Kortas-Stempak, Adrian Strzelecki, Anna Gliwińska, Kamil Dąbkowski, Maciej Jankowski, *Impact of plant-based diet on lipid risk factors for atherosclerosis.* Vol. 23. 2016. 141-148.

101.   *Continuous Update Project Report: Diet, Nutrition, Physical Activity and Colorectal Cancer.* 2017.

102.   Song, M., et al., *Fiber intake and survival after colorectal cancer diagnosis.* JAMA Oncology, 2018. **4**(1): p. 71-79.

103.   Aune, D., et al., *Fruit and vegetable intake and the risk of cardiovascular disease, total cancer and all-cause mortality—a systematic review and dose-response meta-analysis of prospective studies.* International Journal of Epidemiology, 2017. **46**(3): p. 1029-1056.

104.   *USDA Food Composition Databases.* 2017 [cited 2018 January 10, 2018]; Available from: https://ndb.nal.usda.gov/ndb/search/list.

105.   Alonso, A., et al., *Fruit and vegetable consumption is inversely associated with blood pressure in a Mediterranean population with a high vegetable-fat intake: the Seguimiento Universidad de Navarra (SUN) Study.* Br J Nutr, 2004. **92**(2): p. 311-9.

106.   Ornish, D., et al., *Can lifestyle changes reverse coronary heart disease?* The Lancet. **336**(8708): p. 129-133.

107.   Ornish, D., et al., *Intensive lifestyle changes for reversal of coronary heart disease.* Jama, 1998. **280**(23): p. 2001-7.

108.   *Ornish Lifestyle Medicine.* 2018 [cited 2018 January 12, 2018]; Available from: https://www.ornish.com/.

109.   Trichopoulou , A., et al., *Adherence to a Mediterranean Diet and Survival in a Greek Population.* New England Journal of Medicine, 2003. **348**(26): p. 2599-2608.

110.   *Traditional Med Diet.* Available from: https://oldwayspt.org/traditional-diets/mediterranean-diet/traditional-med-diet.

111.   Sacks , F.M., et al., *Effects on Blood Pressure of Reduced Dietary Sodium and the Dietary Approaches to Stop Hypertension (DASH) Diet.* New England Journal of Medicine, 2001. **344**(1): p. 3-10.

112. *Table 1. Top Food Sources of Saturated Fat Among U.S. Population, 2005-2006 NHANES*. 2005-2006 April 20, 2016 March 19, 2018]; Available from: https://epi.grants.cancer.gov/diet/foodsources/sat_fat/sf.html.

113. *Table 5a. Mean Intake of Added Sugars & Percentage Contribution of Various Foods Among U.S. Population, by Age, NHANES 2005-06*. 2016 April 22, 2016 [cited 2018 February 20, 2018]; Available from: https://epi.grants.cancer.gov/diet/foodsources/added_sugars/table5a.html.

114. Gearhardt, A.N., et al., *An Examination of the Food Addiction Construct in Obese Patients with Binge Eating Disorder.* The International Journal of Eating Disorders, 2012. **45**(5): p. 657-663.

115. Bouvard, V., et al., *Carcinogenicity of consumption of red and processed meat.* The Lancet Oncology. **16**(16): p. 1599-1600.

116. Moore, L.V.T., Frances E., *Adults Meeting Fruit and Vegetable Intake Recommendations - United States, 2013*, in *Morbidity and Mortality Weekly Report* 2015. p. 709-713.

117. *Position Paper: Vegetarian Diets.* 2016. p. 1970-1980.

118. Michael, C. and T. David, *Comparative analysis of environmental impacts of agricultural production systems, agricultural input efficiency, and food choice.* Environmental Research Letters, 2017. **12**(6): p. 064016.

119. Global Monitoring Division, E.-G. *CO2 at NOAA's Mauna Loa Observatory reaches new milestone: Tops 400 ppm*. 2013 May 10, 2013 [cited 2018 February 12, 2018]; Available from: https://www.esrl.noaa.gov/gmd/news/7074.html.

120. Gerber, P.J., et al., *Tackling climate change through livestock: a global assessment of emissions and mitigation opportunities*. 2013, Rome: Food and Agriculture Organization of the United Nations (FAO). xxi + 115 pp.

121. *IPCC Fourth Assessment Report: Climate Change 2007* Climate Change 2007: Working Group I: The Physical Science Basis 2007 [cited 2018 February 19, 2018]; Available from: http://www.ipcc.ch/publications_and_data/ar4/wg1/en/ch2s2-10-2.html#table-2-14.

122. Reijnders, L. and S. Soret, *Quantification of the environmental impact of different dietary protein choices.* The American Journal of Clinical Nutrition, 2003. **78**(3): p. 664S-668S.

123. Chadwick, D., et al., *Manure management: Implications for greenhouse gas emissions.* Animal Feed Science and Technology, 2011. **166-167**: p. 514-531.

124. Roll, R., *Scott Harrison, Episode #305*, in *Scott Harrison on Why Clean Water Changes Everything*. 2017, Rich Roll.

125. FAO. *AQUASTAT Water Use by Sector*. 2016; Available from: http://www.fao.org/nr/water/aquastat/water_use/index.stm.

126. Mekonnen, M.M. and A.Y. Hoekstra, *A Global Assessment of the Water Footprint of Farm Animal Products*. Ecosystems, 2012. **15**(3): p. 401-415.

127. Martin, M.J., S.E. Thottathil, and T.B. Newman, *Antibiotics Overuse in Animal Agriculture: A Call to Action for Health Care Providers*. American Journal of Public Health, 2015. **105**(12): p. 2409-2410.

128. Sneeringer, S. *Restrictions on Antibiotic Use for Production Purposes in U.S. Livestock Industries Likely To Have Small Effects on Prices and Quantities*. 2015 November 24, 2015 [cited 2018 February 20, 2018]; Available from: https://www.ers.usda.gov/amber-waves/2015/november/restrictions-on-antibiotic-use-for-production-purposes-in-us-livestock-industries-likely-to-have-small-effects-on-prices-and-quantities/

129. Kreuzig, R. and S. Holtge, *Investigations on the fate of sulfadiazine in manured soil: laboratory experiments and test plot studies*. Environ Toxicol Chem, 2005. **24**(4): p. 771-6.

130. Kümmerer, K., *Antibiotics in the aquatic environment – A review – Part I*. Chemosphere, 2009. **75**(4): p. 417-434.

131. Geist, H.J. and E.F. Lambin, *Proximate Causes and Underlying Driving Forces of Tropical DeforestationTropical forests are disappearing as the result of many pressures, both local and regional, acting in various combinations in different geographical locations*. BioScience, 2002. **52**(2): p. 143-150.

132. Kim, D.-H., J.O. Sexton, and J.R. Townshend, *Accelerated deforestation in the humid tropics from the 1990s to the 2000s*. Geophysical Research Letters, 2015. **42**(9): p. 3495-3501.

133. W. Gay, S. and K. F. Knowlton, *Ammonia Emissions and Animal Agriculture*. 2009.

134. Xiong, X., et al., *Copper content in animal manures and potential risk of soil copper pollution with animal manure use in agriculture*. Resources, Conservation and Recycling, 2010. **54**(11): p. 985-990.

135. Yazdankhah, S., K. Rudi, and A. Bernhoft, *Zinc and copper in animal feed – development of resistance and co-resistance to antimicrobial agents in bacteria of animal origin*. Microbial Ecology in Health and Disease, 2014. **25**: p. 10.3402/mehd.v25.25862.

136. Nagajyoti, P.C., K.D. Lee, and T.V.M. Sreekanth, *Heavy metals, occurrence and toxicity for plants: a review*. Environmental Chemistry Letters, 2010. **8**(3): p. 199-216.

137. Reuther, W., *Copper and Soil Fertility*, in *Yearbook in Agriculture*. 1957: National Agricultural Library Digital Collections. p. 128-135.

138. Tilman, D. and M. Clark, *Global diets link environmental sustainability and human health.* Nature, 2014. **515**(7528): p. 518-22.

139. Aubin, J., *Life Cycle Assessment as applied to environmental choices regarding farmed or wild-caught fish.* CAB Reviews Perspectives in Agriculture Veterinary Science Nutrition and Natural Resources, 2013. **8**(011): p. 1-10.

140. *The State of World Fisheries and Aquaculture.* 2016, FAO. p. 200.

141. Fey, S.B., et al., *Recent shifts in the occurrence, cause, and magnitude of animal mass mortality events.* Proceedings of the National Academy of Sciences, 2015.

142. Mishra, S., et al., *A multicenter randomized controlled trial of a plant-based nutrition program to reduce body weight and cardiovascular risk in the corporate setting: the GEICO study.* European Journal of Clinical Nutrition, 2013. **67**(7): p. 718-724.

143. Goetzel, R.Z., et al., *A multi-worksite analysis of the relationships among body mass index, medical utilization, and worker productivity.* J Occup Environ Med, 2010. **52 Suppl 1**: p. S52-8.

144. Robroek, S.J., et al., *The role of obesity and lifestyle behaviours in a productive workforce.* Occup Environ Med, 2011. **68**(2): p. 134-9.

145. Ricci, J.A. and E. Chee, *Lost productive time associated with excess weight in the U.S. workforce.* J Occup Environ Med, 2005. **47**(12): p. 1227-34.

146. *Lisinopril (Oral route).* Micromedex Detailed Drug Information for the Consumer [Internet]. 2017 [cited 2018 January 5, 2018]; Available from: https://www.ncbi.nlm.nih.gov/pubmedhealth/PMH0046064/#DDIC602023 .side_effects_section.

147. *Number of lisinopril prescriptions in the U.S. from 2004 to 2014 (in millions).* Health & Pharmaceuticals, Pharmaceutical Products & Market 2017 [cited 2018 February 23, 2018]; Available from: https://www.statista.com/statistics/779771/lisinopril-prescriptions-number-in-the-us/.

148. *Part D Drug National Summary Table.* 2017 May 25, 2017 [cited 2018 January 5, 2018]; Available from: https://www.cms.gov/Research-Statistics-Data-and-Systems/Statistics-Trends-and-Reports/Medicare-Provider-Charge-Data/PartD2015.html.

149. Tsai, S.P., et al., *The impact of obesity on illness absence and productivity in an industrial population of petrochemical workers.* Ann Epidemiol, 2008. **18**(1): p. 8-14.

150. Goettler, A., A. Grosse, and D. Sonntag, *Productivity loss due to overweight and obesity: a systematic review of indirect costs.* BMJ Open, 2017. **7**(10).

151. Fallah-Fini, S., et al., *The Additional Costs and Health Effects of a Patient Having Overweight or Obesity: A Computational Model.* Obesity, 2017. **25**(10): p. 1809-1815.

152. *BRFSS Web Enabled Analysis Tool.* 2017 [cited 2018 January 7, 2018]; Available from: https://nccd.cdc.gov/weat/index.html#/crossTabulation/view.

153. Whelan, T.F., Carly, *The Comprehensive Business Case for Sustainability*, in *Harvard Business Review.* 2016, Harvard Business Publishing.

154. Westhoek, H., et al., *Food choices, health and environment: Effects of cutting Europe's meat and dairy intake.* Global environmental change, 2014. **2014 v.26**: p. pp. 196-205.

155. Koruda, E., *More Carrot, Less Stick: Workplace Wellness Programs & The Discriminatory Impact of Financial and Health-Based Incentives.* Boston College Journal of Law & Social Justice, 2016. **36**(1): p. 29.

156. Zajonc, R.B., *Attitudinal effects of mere exposure.* Journal of Personality and Social Psychology, 1968. **9**(2, Pt.2): p. 1-27.

157. Pliner, P., *The Effects of Mere Exposure on Liking for Edible Substances.* Appetite, 1982. **3**(3): p. 283-290.

158. Lakkakula, A., et al., *Repeated taste exposure increases liking for vegetables by low-income elementary school children.* Appetite, 2010. **55**(2): p. 226-31.